EFT for WEIGHT LOSS

The Revolutionary Technique for Conquering
Emotional Overeating, Cravings, Bingeing,
Eating Disorders, and Self-Sabotage

Featuring Reports from EFT Practitioners,
Instructors, Students, and Users

by Gary Craig
www.EFTUniverse.com

Energy Psychology Press
P.O. Box 442, Fulton, CA 95439
www.energypsychologypress.com

Cataloging-in-Publication Data

Craig, Gary, 1940–

EFT for weight loss : the revolutionary technique for conquering emotional overeating, cravings, bingeing, eating disorders, and self-sabotage / by Gary Craig — 1st ed.

p. cm.

"Featuring reports from EFT practitioners, instructors, students, and users."
Includes index.

ISBN 978-1-60415-048-3

1. Weight loss. 2. Emotional Freedom Techniques. 3. Eating disorders—Alternative treatment. I. Title.

RM222.2.C716 2010

613.2'5—dc22

2010028365

Cover design by Victoria Valentine
Editing by CJ Puotinen and Tina Craig
Typesetting by Karin Kinsey
Typeset in Cochin and Adobe Garamond
Printed in USA by Bang Printing
First Edition

10 9 8 7 6 5 4 3 2 1

Important note: While EFT (Emotional Freedom Techniques) has produced remarkable clinical results, it must still be considered to be in the experimental stage and thus practitioners and the public must take complete responsibility for their use of it. Further, Gary Craig is not a licensed health professional and offers EFT as an ordained minister and as a personal performance coach.

Please consult qualified health practitioners regarding your use of EFT.

Contents

A Vital Guide for
Reading This Book

In a nutshell, EFT is an emotional version of acupuncture, except we don't use needles. Instead, we stimulate the acupuncture meridians by tapping on them with our fingertips. This often brings forth astonishing results that are likely beyond your expectations. The procedure is easy to learn and easy to use. You will learn the basics and more in this book.

Because EFT is so versatile, we often say, "Try It on Everything." While this book focuses on EFT's use for weight loss and emotional overeating, I must emphasize that **emotional overeating represents but a tiny fraction of EFT's long list of successes.** For example, EFT is often useful for pain and symptoms of all kinds and often works where nothing else will. It is also astonishingly useful for emotional issues of every type. Further, those wishing to improve their performance in sports, business, public speaking, or the bedroom will also find EFT a valuable aid.

This book is an extensive resource. It is so comprehensive that you might find yourself referring to it over and over again. Most readers will not need to read it all, but every reader will want to keep it around as a priceless resource because it contains approaches and concepts that you will not find in other health-related books.

This book contains creative approaches written by many EFT experts. EFT is an "open source" healing tool that encourages experimentation. This means that we start with an easy-to-learn, simple procedure that works beautifully in the majority of cases. After that, anyone can experiment with the process and develop other refinements. Thus, for your expanded education, we are sprinkling within this book the opinions, refinements, and creative approaches of dozens of EFTers.

Depending on your interest level, previous experience, and individual response to EFT, there are several ways to read this book.

If you are new to EFT, I suggest you start at the beginning and read it all the way through. By the time you reach the end, you will have an excellent chance of being completely and permanently free from out-of-control cravings in addition to having a thorough understanding of EFT and the ability to share this useful technique with friends and family.

If you're interested in the background of EFT and some of the technical, scientific, or engineering explanations that I'm fond of sharing, download our free EFT starter kit from the EFT website, www.EFTUniverse. com. This book was designed as a companion to the main guide to learning EFT, *The EFT Manual,* and you'll learn something valuable from both.

For convenience, a condensed version of the manual is also available as a paperback book sold in retail bookstores and online. Look for *The EFT Manual (EFT: Emotional Freedom Techniques)* by Gary Craig, published by Energy Psychology Press, 2008.

If you're an experienced EFT'er, peruse the Table of Contents and go where your curiosity and interest take you. One of my goals in writing this book is to provide as many interesting examples as possible, so that all of us—including EFT professionals—can add to our repertoire of approaches and strategies for making EFT more effective and versatile.

EFT books and trainings are vital to your complete comprehension of EFT. I would like to emphasize that this book and *The EFT Manual* do not contain everything there is to know about EFT. For example, there is no substitute for the demonstrations in our training seminars, study guides, books, and DVDs.

Once you understand the basics by watching the first few EFT demonstrations, you can get copies of an EFT DVD and then simply tap along. While doing so, you can collapse or neutralize issues that have until now interfered with your weight-loss goals.

EFT professional training and certification is also available. Whether you are already in the healing field, or interested in building an EFT practice, you will find the study guides and the EFT certification process a valuable addition to your therapeutic toolkit. Look for the Certification tab at www.EFTUniverse.com.

Notes and Acknowledgments

The list of individuals who contributed to the development of EFT can never be complete because most of them lived over 5,000 years ago. Those are the brilliant physicians who discovered and mapped the centerpiece of EFT, namely, the subtle energies that course through our bodies. These subtle energies are also the centerpiece of acupuncture and, as a result, EFT and acupuncture are cousins. Both disciplines are growing rapidly here in the West and, as time unfolds, they are destined to have a primary role in emotional and physical healing.

In the 20th Century, other dedicated souls advanced our use of ancient techniques that utilize the body's energy. Principal among them is Dr. George Goodheart, who developed Applied Kinesiology, a forerunner of EFT. In the 1960s, Dr. Goodheart discovered that muscle testing could be used to gather important information from the body, and he went on to train many health care practitioners and publish important books and papers.

Dr. John Diamond's work deserves applause because, to my knowledge, he was one of the first psychiatrists to use and write about these subtle energies. His many pioneering concepts, together with advanced ideas from Applied Kinesiology, have formed the foundation upon which our work is constructed. Dr. Diamond's best-sellers include *Life Energy: Using the Meridians to Unlock the Power of Your Emotions* (Continuum International, 1990) and *Life Energy and the Emotions* (Eden Grove, 1997).

Dr. Roger Callahan, the clinical psychologist from whom I received my original introduction to "emotional acupressure," deserves all the credit history can give him. He was the first to bring these techniques to the public in a substantial way and he did so despite open hostility from his own profession. As you might appreciate, it takes heavy doses of conviction to plow through the ingrained beliefs of conventional thinking. Without Roger Callahan's missionary drive, we might still be sitting around theorizing about this "interesting thing."

It is upon the shoulders of these giants that I humbly stand. My own contribution to the rapidly expanding field of meridian therapies has been to reduce the unnecessary complexity that inevitably finds its way into new discoveries. EFT is an elegantly simple version of these procedures, which professionals and laypeople alike can use on a variety of problems.

I also owe a special debt of gratitude to Adrienne Fowlie, who, through a friend, introduced me to meridian tapping techniques and helped me develop EFT.

Many EFT students and practitioners helped make this book possible. I am grateful to all who contributed case studies and reports. Most of the examples given here were published in our email newsletter and are posted in the newsletter's archives at the EFT website, www.EFTUniverse.com. The growth of this collection of reports has been something to behold. Awesome is an appropriate word, as there are so many articles in this collection that they could be bound into personalized reference books on many topics. Our website is loaded with some of the best of these contributions.

The names given in the reports presented here have often been changed to protect the privacy of those involved. This is especially likely if only first names are given. When a person's full name is given, it has not been changed and is used with permission.

In the interests of editorial consistency, reports from the United Kingdom, Australia, Canada, and other countries that use British spelling and punctuation have been changed to conform to standard American English.

Like most topics of special interest, EFT has its own language, words, or abbreviations that have special meaning for its students and practitioners. You'll find a list of EFT terms and their definitions in the Glossary.

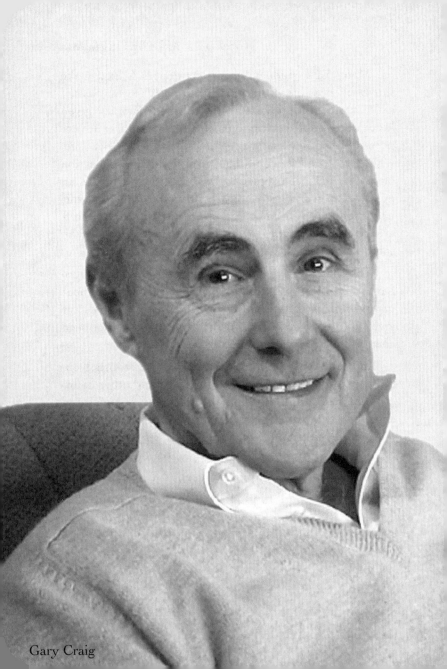
Gary Craig

Introduction

Are you overeating as a way to suppress or soothe uncomfortable emotions, such as stress, anger, anxiety, boredom, sadness, and loneliness? If so, you may be an emotional overeater.

Obesity has reached epidemic proportions in the United States, and at any given time, about half of America's women and a quarter of its men are on a diet. Dieting has grown to a $40-billion-a-year industry at the same time most dieters are failing. It is estimated that 95 percent of successful dieters gain their lost weight back within five years.

Recently, celebrities like Oprah Winfrey and Dr. Phil McGraw have brought attention to emotional overeating, but the standard advice of trying talk therapy, journaling, and keeping a food/mood diary in addition to counting calories, carbohydrates, and fat grams doesn't seem to work for many.

That personal work can be a step in the right direction because it helps people tune into their reasons for overeating, *but there is something more subtle at the root of emotional eating.* Unresolved emotional issues or traumas create blocks or disruptions in the body's subtle energy systems. *These energy disruptions create a type of "anxiety short circuit" in the body that, in turn, triggers overeating.* This overeating serves to calm anxiety, but at the expense of consuming unnecessary calories.

EFT is a highly effective aid to weight loss because it is very relaxing and usually removes anxiety. With the anxiety gone, the drive for emotional overeating disappears. Further, EFT helps to reprogram your energy system so that you eat for nutrition rather than to tranquilize emotions.

EFT helps people resolve their emotional issues because it addresses energy imbalances that are so often behind one's unresolved negative emotions.

Have you ever found anything that takes away your cravings for junk food? Other than giving in and eating the food you were craving, that is! Cravings happen to just about everyone. It's what we do when they hit that makes all the difference.

Cravings are often a result of our emotions, anxiety, or stress. Our bodies crave high-sugar, high-fat foods as a way to "medicate" ourselves into a calmer state when we are avoiding our emotions or under a lot of stress. When we are in emotionally stressful states, our bodies' energy flow may be blocked or reversed.

Did you know you can totally eliminate food cravings in seconds? You'll find step-by-step instructions and numerous examples for getting rid of cravings in this book.

Your job on this weight-loss path isn't just about losing weight. It's about making a mental turnaround so that your weight loss is permanent. Part of the reason many people gain back their lost weight is because their mental outlook never changed. *Change your perspective and you will change your life.*

Of course, this is easier said than done. If New Year's resolutions always worked, we'd all be perfect. Resolutions to change our habits, change our thoughts, and change our bodies all hit the same enormous bump in the road, and that's self-sabotage.

What causes self-sabotage? That's simple — it's caused by the same energy blocks that contribute to negative thoughts and uncomfortable physical symptoms. Because EFT addresses the underlying causes of energy blocks and all of their manifestations, it is a powerful tool that anyone can use to make powerful, permanent changes.

Whether you are new to EFT or already an experienced tapper, I am very pleased to share this book with you. I know without a doubt that EFT can help you take control of your health and happiness and that the instructions and recommendations given here can completely transform not only your weight but your entire life.

1

EFT's Basic Recipe
by Gary Craig

The basic premise of the Emotional Freedom Techniques is *that the cause of all negative emotions is a disruption in the body's energy system.* In EFT this premise is termed the "Discovery Statement," and I can't emphasize this concept enough. When our energy is flowing normally, without obstruction, we feel good in every way. When our energy becomes blocked or stagnant or is otherwise disrupted along one or more of the body's energy meridians, negative or damaging emotions can develop along with all types of physical symptoms. This idea has been the centerpiece of Eastern medicine for thousands of years.

EFT is often called *emotional acupuncture* because it combines gentle tapping on key acupuncture points while focusing your thoughts on pain, unhappy memories, uncomfortable emotions, food cravings, or any other problem. When properly done, the underlying emotional

factors that contribute to the problem are typically released along with the energy blocks.

Consider that:

EFT often works when nothing else will.

*Further, it can bring complete or partial relief in about
80 percent of the cases* in which it's tried, and in the hands
of a skilled practitioner, its success rate can exceed 95
percent.

Sometimes the improvement is permanent, while in other
cases the process needs to be continued. But even if symptoms return, they can usually be reduced or eliminated
quickly and effectively just by repeating the procedure.

*People are often astonished at the results they experience
because their belief systems have not yet adapted to this common-
sense process.* The treatment of physical, emotional, and
performance issues is supposed to be much more difficult
than simply tapping with your fingertips on key acupuncture points.

The EFT basics are extremely easy to use. Small children
learn it quickly, and kids as young as eight or ten have no
trouble teaching it to others. It's fully portable, requires
no special equipment, and can be used at any time of the
day or night and under any circumstances.

*No drugs, surgeries, radiations, or other medical interven-
tions* are involved in EFT. In fact, it's so different from
conventional medicine that the medical profession often
has difficulty explaining its results.

It doesn't seem to matter what the patient's blood tests
or other diagnostic tests show. *Relief can occur with EFT*

no matter what your diagnosis. That's because we are addressing a different cause that tends to be outside the medical box.

This is not to say you should ignore your physician's advice. On the contrary, I encourage you to *consult with qualified health-care providers.* Quite a few EFT practitioners are physicians, nurses, dentists, acupuncturists, chiropractors, massage therapists, psychologists, counselors, and other health-care professionals. As EFT becomes more widely known, it will become easier to find licensed health-care providers who are knowledgeable about EFT.

Using a few minutes of EFT will often improve your physical health. When it doesn't, there is likely to be some *underlying emotional issue* that is creating chemicals and/ or tension in your body, which can interfere with your success.

If that's the case, *EFT is ideal for collapsing and neutralizing emotional issues* and it often does the job in minutes. EFT was originally designed for reducing the psychotherapy process from months or years down to minutes or, in complicated cases, a few sessions.

No technique or procedure works for everyone, but by all accounts the vast majority of those who try EFT for a specific problem experience significant improvement. That's a stunning result and one that compares favorably with prescription drugs, surgical procedures, and other medical treatments. I encourage practitioners and newcomers alike to experiment—to try it on everything. It makes sense that if your energy is balanced, everything inside and around you benefits.

Whether you are new to EFT or already an experienced tapper, I am very pleased to share this information with you. I know without a doubt that EFT can help you take control of your health and happiness and that the instructions and recommendations given here can completely transform your life.

Defining the Problem

EFT sessions usually begin with a self-estimate of discomfort using a scale from 0 to 10. We call this the 0-to-10 intensity meter or intensity scale. The discomfort being measured can be physical, such as headache pain or a craving, or it can be an emotion such as fear, anxiety, depression, or anger.

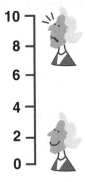

Intensity Meter

It's a good idea to rate every problem before and after you apply EFT so that you can determine how much progress you're making. It's also important to assess your intensity as it exists now rather than when the event or problem first occurred.

Don't worry if you find it difficult to select a specific number—sometimes newbies (my affectionate term for EFT newcomers) get distracted by this part of the procedure and worry unnecessarily about whether it's a 5 or a 6, or a 2 or a 3. Using the 10-point scale becomes easy with practice. Just give yourself a number to get started and it will soon be automatic. It helps to remind yourself that there are no wrong answers here and that if you have trouble coming up with a specific number, a guess will work fine. It is simply a benchmark for comparison before and after you perform EFT.

For reference, jot the number down and add a few notes. For example, if you're focusing on a pain, think about where the pain is located, how it interferes with your range of motion, and whether it hurts more when you move to the left or right, stand or sit, and so forth.

Another way to indicate the intensity of pain or discomfort, which works well for children, is to stretch one's arms wide apart for major pain and bring them close together for minor pain. Some children find it easier to express "big" and "small" with their hands than with a number scale.

The method you choose doesn't matter as long as it works for you. Keeping track of your pain's intensity before and after treatment is the easiest way to determine whether and how effectively the treatment is working.

The same scale works for feelings. First, focus on an event or memory or problem that has been bothering you. Now ask yourself how angry, anxious, depressed, or upset are you on a scale from 0 to 10. If it doesn't bother you at all, you're at 0. If you're at 10, that's the most it has ever been. Get in the habit of starting each tapping session with an intensity measurement and make a note of it.

Now I'd like to introduce you to the Basic Recipe, the formula that is the foundation of this technique.

The Basic Recipe

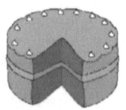

A recipe has certain ingredients that must be added in a certain order. If you are baking a cake, for example, you must use sugar instead of pepper and you must add the sugar before you put it in the oven. Otherwise... no cake.

Basic EFT is like a cake recipe. It has specific ingredients that go together in a specific way. Just as someone who is learning to cook will get best results from following tried and true instructions, someone who is new to EFT will do well to learn the Basic Recipe. An accomplished chef will take a different approach, and so can you once you master the fundamentals.

What I'm going to show you here is a shortcut method of using EFT. It does not include everything that I teach in the many other EFT training resources. It also omits a process called the 9 Gamut Procedure that was part of the earliest version of EFT. The Full Basic Recipe includes the 9 Gamut Procedure, which can be highly useful. After developing EFT, however, I discovered that this shortcut method works very well almost all of the time, so this is the primary method I now use, and so do most EFT practitioners. I encourage everyone to learn or at least know about the original version so that if you don't get the results you want, you can try the Full Basic Recipe (see Appendix A). It is easy to learn and adds less than a minute to the procedure.

Focusing now on the shortcut method, here is what you need in order to start using EFT.

Ingredient #1: The Setup

Applying the Basic Recipe is something like going bowling. In bowling, there is a machine that sets up the pins by picking them up and arranging them in perfect order at the end of the alley. Once this "setup" is done, all you need to do is roll the ball down the alley to knock over the pins.

In a similar manner, the Basic Recipe has a beginning routine to "set up" your energy system as though it is a set of bowling pins. This routine (called the Setup) is vital to the whole process and prepares the energy system so that the rest of the Basic Recipe (the ball) can do its job.

Your energy system, of course, is not *really* a set of bowling pins. It is a set of subtle electric circuits. I present this bowling analogy only to give you a sense of the purpose of the Setup and the need to *make sure your energy system is properly oriented before attempting to remove its disruptions.*

Your energy system is subject to a form of electrical interference that can block the balancing effect of these tapping procedures. When present, this interfering block-age must be removed or the Basic Recipe will not work. Removing it is the job of the Setup.

Technically speaking, this interfering blockage takes the form of a *polarity reversal* within your energy system. This is different from the *energy disruptions* that cause your negative emotions.

Another analogy may help us here. Consider a flash-light or any other device that runs on batteries. If the batteries aren't there, it won't work. Equally important, the batteries must be installed properly. You've noticed, I'm sure, that batteries have + and - marks on them. These marks indicate their polarity. If you line up the + and - marks according to the instructions, the electricity flows normally and your flashlight works fine.

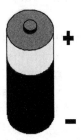

But what happens if you put the batteries in back-ward? Try it sometime. The flashlight will not work. It acts as if the batteries have been removed. That's what happens when polarity reversal is present in your energy system. It's as though your batteries are in backward. I don't mean that you stop working altogether—like turn "toes up" and die—but your progress does become arrested in some areas.

Psychological Reversal

This polarity reversal has an official name. It is called Psychological Reversal and it represents a fascinating discovery with wide-ranging applications in all areas of healing and personal performance.

It is the reason why some diseases are chronic and respond very poorly to conventional treatments. It is the reason why some people have such a difficult time losing weight or giving up addictive substances. It is also the reason why talented athletes "freeze" or make game-losing mistakes or never achieve their full potential. It is, quite literally, the cause of self-sabotage.

Psychological Reversal is caused by self-defeating, negative thinking that often occurs subconsciously and thus outside of your awareness. On average, it will be present—and thus hinder EFT—about 40 percent of the time. Some people have very little of it (this is rare) while others are beset by it most of the time (this also is rare). Most people fall somewhere in between these two extremes. Psychological Reversal doesn't create any feelings within you, so you won't know if it is present or not. Even the most positive people are subject to it…including yours truly.

When Psychological Reversal is present, it will stop any attempt at healing, including EFT, dead in its tracks. Therefore it *must* be corrected if the rest of the Basic Recipe is going to work.

We correct for Psychological Reversal even though it might not be present. It only takes 8 or 10 seconds to do and, if it isn't present, no harm is done. If it is present, however, a major impediment to your success will be out of the way.

The Setup consists of two parts:

1. Saying an affirmation three times while
2. Correcting simultaneously for Psychological Reversal.

The Affirmation

Since the cause of Psychological Reversal involves negative thinking, it should come as no surprise that the correction for it includes a neutralizing affirmation. Such is the case with EFT, and here it is:

> *Even though I have this _____, I deeply and completely accept myself.*

Fill in the blank with a brief description of the problem you want to address. Here are some examples.

> *Even though I have this <u>pain in my lower back</u>, I deeply and completely accept myself.*

> *Even though I have this <u>fear of public speaking</u>, I deeply and completely accept myself.*

> *Even though I have this <u>headache</u>, I deeply and completely accept myself.*

Even though I have this <u>anger toward my father</u>, I deeply and completely accept myself.

Even though I have this <u>war memory</u>, I deeply and completely accept myself.

Even though I have this <u>stiffness in my neck</u>, I deeply and completely accept myself.

Even though I have these <u>nightmares</u>, I deeply and completely accept myself.

Even though I have this <u>craving for chocolate</u>, I deeply and completely accept myself.

Even though I have this <u>fear of snakes</u>, I deeply and completely accept myself.

This is only a partial list, of course, because the possible issues that are addressable by EFT are endless. You can also vary the Acceptance Phrase by saying:

"I accept myself even though I have this _____."

"Even though I have this _____, I deeply and profoundly accept myself."

"Even though I have this _____, I love and forgive myself."

"I love and accept myself even though I have this _____."

And there are more variations. Instead of saying, "I deeply and completely accept myself," you can simply say:

I'm okay.   *I'll be okay.*

I'll feel better soon.   *Everything's improving.*

Or something similar. This, by the way, is how we use EFT with children. The phrase "I deeply and completely accept myself" makes little sense to kids. Instead, a child who's upset can say something like the following:

Even though I flunked the math test, I'm a cool kid, I'm okay.

Even though I lost my backpack and I'm mad at myself, I'm still an awesome kid.

All of these affirmations are correct because they follow the same general format. That is, they acknowledge the problem and create self-acceptance despite the existence of the problem.

That's what is necessary for the affirmation to be effective. You can use any version, but I suggest you start with the recommended one because it is easy to memorize and has a good track record of getting the job done.

Now here are some interesting points about the affirmation.

- It doesn't matter whether you believe the affirmation or not. Just say it.

- It is better to say it with feeling and emphasis, but saying it routinely will usually do the job.

- It is best to say it out loud, but if you are in a social situation where you prefer to mutter it under your breath or do it silently, then go ahead. It will probably be effective.

Correcting for Psychological Reversal

To add to the effectiveness of the affirmation, the Setup includes a simple method for clearing Psychological Reversal. You do this by tapping the Karate Chop point, which is explained next, while reciting the affirmation.

The Karate Chop Point

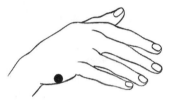

The Karate Chop (KC) Point

The Karate Chop point (abbreviated **KC**) is located at the center of the fleshy part of the outside of your hand (either hand) between the top of the wrist and the base of the baby finger—or, stated differently, the part of your hand you would use to deliver a karate chop.

Tap the Karate Chop point solidly with the tips of the index finger and middle finger—or all four fingers—of the opposite hand. Although you can use the Karate Chop point of either hand, it is usually most convenient to tap the Karate Chop point of the nondominant hand with the fingertips of the dominant hand. If you are right-handed, tap the Karate Chop point on your left hand with the fingertips of your right hand. If you are left-handed, tap the Karate Chop point on your right hand with the fingertips of your left hand.

Now that you understand the parts of the Setup, performing it is easy. You create a word or short phrase to fill in the blank in the affirmation and then simply *repeat the affirmation, with emphasis, three times while continuously tapping the Karate Chop point.*

That's it. After a few practice rounds, you should be able to perform the Setup in 8 to 10 seconds or so. Now, with the Setup properly performed, you are ready for the next ingredient in the Basic Recipe: the Sequence.

Ingredient #2: The Sequence

The Sequence is simple in concept. It involves tapping at or near the end points of the body's major energy flows, which are called *meridians* in traditional Chinese medicine, and it is the method by which the disruption in the energy system is corrected or balanced. Before locating these points, however, you need a few tips on how to carry out the tapping process.

Tapping tips:

- You can tap with either hand, but it is usually more convenient to do so with your dominant hand (your right hand if you are right-handed or your left hand if you are left-handed).

- Tap with the fingertips of your index finger and middle finger. This covers a little larger area than just tapping with one fingertip and allows you to cover the tapping points more easily.

- Tap solidly but never so hard as to hurt or bruise yourself.

- Tap about seven times on each of the tapping points. I say *about* seven times because you will be repeating a "Reminder Phrase" (explained later) while tapping and it will be difficult to count at the same time. If you are a little over or a little under seven (five to nine, for example) that will be sufficient.

Most of the tapping points exist on both sides of the body. It doesn't matter which side you use nor does it matter if you switch sides during the Sequence. For example, you can tap under your right eye and, later in the Sequence, tap under your left arm.

The points:

Each energy meridian has two end points. For the purposes of the Basic Recipe, you need only tap on one end point to balance out any disruptions that may exist in the meridian. These end points are near the surface of the body and are thus more readily accessed than other points along the meridians that may be more deeply buried. What follows are instructions on how to locate the end points of those meridians that are important to the Basic Recipe. Taken together and tapped in the order presented, they form the Sequence.

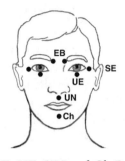

EB, SE, UE, UN and Ch Points

1. **Eyebrow:** At the beginning of the eyebrow, just above and to one side of the nose. This point is abbreviated **EB** for beginning of the Eye**B**row.

2. **Side of Eye:** On the bone bordering the outside corner of the eye. This point is abbreviated **SE** for **S**ide of the **E**ye.

3. **Under Eye:** On the bone under an eye about 1 inch below the pupil. This point is abbreviated **UE** for **U**nder the **E**ye.

4. **Under Nose:** On the small area between the bottom of the nose and the top of the upper lip. This point is abbreviated **UN** for **U**nder the **N**ose.

5. **Chin:** Midway between the point of the chin and the bottom of the lower lip. Although it is not directly on the point of the chin, we call it the Chin Point because it is descriptive enough for people to understand easily. This point is abbreviated **Ch** for **Ch**in.

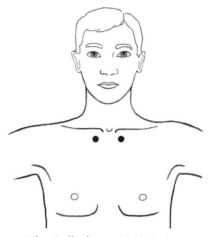

The Collarbone (CB) Points

6. **Collarbone:** The junction where the sternum (breastbone), collarbone, and first rib meet. Place your forefinger on the U-shaped notch at the top of the breastbone (where a man would knot his tie). Move down toward the navel 1 inch and then go to the left (or right) about 1 or 2 inches. This point is abbreviated **CB** for **C**ollar**B**one *even though it is not on the collarbone (or clavicle) per se*. It is at the *beginning* of the collarbone.

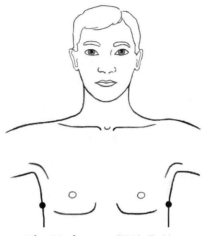

The Underarm (UA) Points

7. **Underarm:** On the side of the body, at a point even with the nipple (for men) or in the middle of the bra strap (for women). It is about 4 inches below the armpit. This point is abbreviated **UA** for **U**nder the **A**rm.

The abbreviations for these points are summarized below in the same order as the previous.

1. **EB** = Beginning of the **E**ye**B**row
2. **SE** = **S**ide of the **E**ye
3. **UE** = **U**nder the **E**ye
4. **UN** = **U**nder the **N**ose
5. **Ch** = **Ch**in
6. **CB** = Beginning of the **C**ollar**B**one
7. **UA** = **U**nder the **A**rm

Please notice that these tapping points proceed *down the body*. That is, each tapping point is *below* the one before it. That should make it a snap to memorize. A few trips through it and it should be yours forever.

The Reminder Phrase

Once memorized, the Basic Recipe becomes a life-time friend. It can be applied to an almost endless list of emotional and physical problems, and it provides relief from most of them. However, there's one more concept we need to develop before we can apply the Basic Recipe to a given problem. It's called the Reminder Phrase.

When a football quarterback throws a pass, he aims it at a particular receiver. He doesn't just throw the ball in the air and hope someone will catch it. Likewise, the Basic Recipe needs to be aimed at a specific problem. Otherwise, it will bounce around aimlessly with little or no effect.

You "aim" the Basic Recipe by applying it while tuned in to the problem from which you want relief. This tells your system which problem needs to be the "receiver."

Remember the EFT discovery statement, which says: *The cause of all negative emotions is a disruption in the body's energy system.*

Negative emotions come about because you are tuned in to certain thoughts or circumstances that, in turn, disrupt your energy system. Otherwise, you function normally. Your fear of heights is not present, for example, while you are reading the comic section of the Sunday newspaper and therefore not tuned in to the problem.

Tuning in to a problem can be done simply by thinking about it. In fact, tuning in *means* thinking about it. Thinking about the problem will bring about the energy disruptions involved, which then, and only then, can be balanced by applying the Basic Recipe. Without tuning in to the problem—thereby creating those energy disruptions—the Basic Recipe does nothing.

Tuning in is seemingly a simple process. You merely think about the problem while applying the Basic Recipe. That's it, at least in theory.

However, you may find it a bit difficult to think consciously about the problem while you are tapping. That's why I'm introducing a Reminder Phrase that you can repeat continually while performing the Basic Recipe.

The Reminder Phrase is a word or short phrase that describes the problem and that you repeat out loud each time you tap one of the points in the Sequence. In this way, you continually "remind" your system about the problem you are working on.

The best Reminder Phrase to use is usually identical to what you choose for the affirmation part of the Setup. For example, if you are working on a fear of public speaking, the Setup affirmation would go like this:

Even though I have this fear of public speaking, I deeply and completely accept myself.

Within this affirmation, the underlined words, *fear of public speaking,* are ideal for use as the Reminder Phrase.

I sometimes use a shorter version of this Reminder Phrase when in seminars. I might, for example, use "public speaking fear" or just "public speaking" instead of the somewhat longer version. That's just one of the shortcuts we have grown accustomed to after years of experience with these techniques. For your purposes, however, you can simply use identical words for both the Setup's affirmation and the Reminder Phrase. That way you will minimize any possibility of error.

Now here's an interesting point: I don't always have people repeat a Reminder Phrase. That's because I have discovered over time that simply stating the affirmation during the Setup is usually sufficient to "tune in" to the problem at hand. The subconscious mind usually locks on to the problem throughout the Basic Recipe even though tapping might seem distracting.

But this is not always true and, with extensive training and experience, one can recognize whether using the Reminder Phrase is necessary. It is not usually necessary, but when it is necessary, it is *really* necessary and must be used.

What's beautiful about EFT is that you don't need to have my experience in this regard. You don't have to be able to figure out whether or not the Reminder Phrase is necessary. You can just *assume* it is always necessary and thereby assure yourself of always being tuned in to the problem by simply repeating the Reminder Phrase as instructed. It does no harm to repeat the Reminder Phrase when it is not necessary, and it will serve as an invaluable tool when it is. We do many things in each round of the Basic Recipe that may not be necessary for a given problem. But when a particular part of the Basic Recipe *is* necessary, *it is absolutely critical.*

It does no harm to include everything, even what may not be needed, and it only takes one minute per round. This includes repeating the Reminder Phrase each time you tap a point during the Sequence. It costs nothing to include it, not even time, because it can be repeated within the same time it takes to tap each energy point seven times.

The Reminder Phrase concept is an easy one. Just to be complete, however, I am including a few samples of the Reminder Phrase:

headache

anger toward my father

war memory

stiffness in my neck

nightmares

craving for chocolate

fear of snakes

Test Your Results

At the end of one or two rounds of tapping all of the points in the Sequence, take another look at the problem you're working on. Measure it on the 0-to-10 intensity scale. Where is it now? You'll be able to test some problems or conditions right away, in the comfort of your living room. Others you'll want to test in the actual settings where they occur.

If the problem doesn't bother you at all anymore and is at 0, congratulations! You're done. No further tapping is required.

If you feel better, but the problem is still there, make a note of your new level of discomfort on the 0-to-10 intensity scale. For example, your headache pain may have gone from a 9 to a 4, or your anger toward your father might have moved from an 8 to a 5. Keeping track of the numbers helps you track your progress.

If you are a practitioner, write down the problem your client is working on, the beginning intensity level, and the level after treatment. This helps both of you appreciate whatever improvement is being made, and it simplifies follow-up sessions.

If you're working on your own, write down every problem or issue you tap for along with your results. Review your notes after a few weeks of practice and you will be amazed at the number of issues you have cleared away, many of which you will have forgotten about by then.

Here's what to do if you or your client still have some discomfort after an initial round of tapping.

Subsequent Round Adjustments

When EFT tapping produces only partial relief, you will need to do one or more additional rounds.

Those subsequent rounds have to be adjusted slightly for best results. Here's why. The first round doesn't always completely eliminate a problem because of the reemergence of Psychological Reversal, that interfering blockage that the Setup is designed to correct.

This time, Psychological Reversal shows up in a somewhat different form. Instead of blocking your progress altogether, it now blocks any *remaining* progress. You make some headway but become stopped on the way to complete relief because Psychological Reversal enters in a manner that keeps you from getting better still.

Since the subconscious mind tends to be literal, subsequent rounds of the Basic Recipe need to address the fact that you are working on the *remaining problem.* Accordingly, the affirmation contained within the Setup has to be adjusted, as does the Reminder Phrase.

> *Even though I **still** have **some** of this* _____, *I deeply and completely accept myself.*

Please note the emphasized words "still" and "some" and how they change the thrust of the affirmation toward the *remainder* of the problem. It should be easy to make this adjustment and, after a little experience, you will fall into it quite naturally.

Study the following affirmations. They reflect adjustments to the sample affirmations earlier in this section.

> *Even though I **still** have **some** of this <u>headache</u>, I deeply and completely accept myself.*

> *Even though I **still** have **some**e of this <u>anger toward my father</u>, I deeply and completely accept myself.*

> *Even though I **still** have **some** of this <u>war memory</u>, I deeply and completely accept myself.*

> *Even though I **still** have **some** of this <u>stiffness in my neck</u>, I deeply and completely accept myself.*

The Reminder Phrase is also easily adjusted. Just put the word "remaining" before the previously used phrase. Here are examples, using the previous Reminder Phrases:

remaining *headache*

remaining *anger toward my father*

remaining *war memory*

remaining *stiffness in my neck*

If your symptom or condition disappears but then returns, simply repeat EFT's Basic Recipe and the "remaining" Reminder Phrase, as described here.

Tapping with and for Others

I should add that EFT can be done by you on yourself, by another person on you, and by you on another person. All of these approaches to EFT tapping work equally well. If you watch my EFT sessions on www.YouTube.com, you will see that in seminars and workshops, I routinely tap on the EFT points of the people I work with onstage. The technique of tapping on another person makes it easy for parents to apply EFT to their infants and small children and for anyone to apply EFT to those who for various reasons are not able to tap on or for themselves.

Introducing Aspects

Aspects are the various pieces of an emotional issue that may show up during an EFT session. Fortunately, they can be handled easily.

For example, let's say you have a fear of spiders that you would like to put behind you. If there is no spider present to cause you any emotional intensity, then close your eyes and imagine seeing a spider, or imagine a past time when a spider scared you. Assess your intensity on a scale of 0 to 10 *as it exists NOW while you think about it.* If you estimate it at a 7, for example, then you have a benchmark against which to measure your progress.

Now do one round of the Basic Recipe and imagine the spider again. If you can find no trace whatsoever of your previous emotional intensity, then you are done. If, on the other hand, you go to, let's say, a 4, then you need to perform subsequent rounds until your intensity falls to 0.

You might wonder at this point whether getting to 0 while just thinking about a spider will hold up when you actually confront a real spider. The answer is usually yes! In most cases, the energy disruptions that occur while thinking about the spider are the same as those that occur when you are in the presence of a real spider. That's why the original energy balancing tends to hold in real circumstances.

The exception to this is when some new aspect of the problem comes up in the real situation that wasn't there when you were just thinking about it. For example, you may have been thinking about a spider that didn't move. If movement is an important aspect of your fear and if it was absent from your thinking when the original EFT rounds were done, then that part of the fear will arise when you see a moving spider.

This is a reasonably common occurrence, and it doesn't mean that EFT didn't work. It simply means there is more to do. Just apply the Basic Recipe to the new aspect (moving spider) until your emotional response falls to 0. Once all aspects have been eliminated, your phobic response to spiders should be history and you can be perfectly calm around them.

Someone who's haunted by a traffic accident might be affected by memories of oncoming headlights, anger toward the other driver, the sound of screeching brakes, or the sight of window glass shattering. A war trauma can have aspects such as the sight of blood, the look in a comrade's eyes before he dies, the sound of a hand grenade, or the memory of an explosion or gunfire. A rape experience can have aspects such as the smell of the assailant's breath, the sound of his voice, the impact of a fist, or the penetration. A fear of public speaking can have aspects such as the sight of a microphone, the observing eyes of the audience, or a memory of being ridiculed as a child.

Another thing to recognize is that an aspect can also be an emotion. Anger regarding a given event may shift to sadness. Pick up on these clues. These different emotional aspects are taking you deeper into the problem. They are opportunities for greater healing and present you with great possibilities for mastering your craft.

The notion of aspects is an important one in EFT. As in the previous examples, some problems have many pieces or aspects to them and the problem will not be completely relieved until all of them are addressed. Actually, each of these aspects qualifies as a separate problem even though they seem to be lumped together. The fear of a stationary spider and the fear of a moving spider, for example, may seem to be one problem. In fact, they may be separate problems that need to be addressed separately with EFT.

Different aspects are possible with just about any problem you want to address with EFT. Each aspect may be a separate problem that needs to be addressed individually before complete relief is obtained.

Please understand that where several aspects of an emotional problem are present, you may not notice any relief until all aspects are reduced to 0 by the Basic Recipe. This becomes very clear when you consider different aspects of physical healing. If, for example, you have a simultaneous headache, toothache, and stomachache, you will not feel healthy until all three are gone. The pain may seem to shift, but it is, nonetheless, still pain. So it is with emotional issues that contain different aspects. Even if you have taken care of one or more aspects, you may not experience relief until all of the problem's aspects have been dealt with.

Experienced EFTers often compare this procedure to peeling an onion. You get rid of one layer only to discover another. When a problem has many layers or aspects, neutralizing them with EFT can seem like a daunting project. But considering how quickly those layers can be dealt with and how beneficial the results are, the project is more exciting than intimidating. And the rewards are priceless.

Core Issues

By far the fastest way to resolve a complex issue or clear up symptoms that resist treatment is to discover the problem's *core issue*. Core issues are fundamental emotional disruptions that can be formed in childhood or in response to a difficult or traumatic event.

In some cases, they are obvious. When asked about when a problem started or what might be contributing to it, the reply is immediate. "I'll bet it has something to do with my husband's heart attack last fall." "I turn to food whenever I think about my wife's affair, and my overeating is out of control." "Ever since my business failed, my back has been killing me."

But many times, core issues are hidden from view. This is because the subconscious mind is a clever protector of secrets, especially those that we hide from ourselves.

In some cases, our subconscious minds hide secrets that are truly awful. But most self-sabotaging secrets, when looked at objectively, don't amount to much.

The reason Tom can't give a presentation at work is because, in fourth grade, his teacher embarrassed him in front of the class. The reason Ann can't lose weight is because, when she was eight years old, her mother told her she would always be too fat to wear a swimsuit. The reason John can't propose to Marie is because his older sister always told him that he was such a loser, no one would ever marry him. The reason Susan can't take an elevator is because when she was trapped in one for five minutes several years ago, the friend who was with her started screaming.

As long as they hold an emotional charge, these secrets are powerful enough to shape a person's life. But as soon as they are uncovered and neutralized with EFT, core issues like these lose their power and become insignificant old memories.

This feature of EFT never ceases to amaze me. Again and again I've worked with people while they dealt with incredibly painful memories, memories that controlled their lives and dictated where they would live, what career they would follow, what friends they would have, and everything else. Suddenly, after a few rounds of EFT tapping, they are completely transformed and no longer frightened, anxious, or afraid of old events. Instead, they're able to describe past traumas as easily as if they are talking about the weather. As soon as old events and old memories lose their emotional charge, they lose their place of power in the subconscious mind.

Be Specific

If you want fast, impressive results with EFT, be specific. Vague statements generate vague outcomes. The biggest mistake made by newcomers is using EFT on issues that are too global. Global problems are broad, vague, or hazy. They aren't well defined. Even with persistence, which can almost always make a difference, global statements are less likely to produce results than specific statements about specific events.

I have been beating the drum for many years about being specific with EFT, urging EFTers to break emotional issues into the events that underlie them. When we do this, we address true causes and not just symptoms. Although there is a skill to doing this, those who take this approach have watched their success rates climb impressively. They are also doing deeper, more meaningful work.

Many newcomers to EFT present their emotional issues in global terms. They say things like:

I feel abandoned. I'm always anxious.

I was an abused child. I hate my father.

I have low self-esteem. I can't do anything right.

I'm depressed. I feel overwhelmed.

To them, that is the problem and that is what they want EFT to fix.

But, despite the person's perception, that is not the problem at all. Those feelings are merely symptoms of the problem. The real problem is the unresolved specific events, memories, and emotions that cause the larger issue. How can one feel abandoned or abused, for example, unless specific events occurred in one's life to cause those feelings? The feelings didn't just appear out of the blue. They must have had a cause.

If we consider the larger issue (such as abandonment) to be a tabletop, then the table's legs represent specific events that support the table (my mother died when I was seven; my father walked out on us when I was eleven; I got lost on a hiking trip in the Sierra Mountains).

Obviously, if we reduce an issue to the specific events supporting it and then collapse its table legs, the tabletop will fall for lack of support. In this way, we address the true causes (specific events and emotions linked to them) rather than just symptoms.

Unfortunately, many EFT practitioners still apply EFT to the tabletop and not the supporting table legs. Thus they might start with:

Even though I have this feeling of abandonment…

Being global like this is the number-one error made by new EFTers and some seasoned ones, too. Interestingly, this approach will sometimes get results, but it is not nearly as thorough or precise as going for the supporting table legs first.

Also, because this global approach lacks precision, those using it are more likely to report that their issues "come back." What "come back," of course, are unresolved events (table legs) that were not previously addressed.

In addition, approaching an issue in a vague or global manner creates an environment in which the person's attention shifts from event to event. You can be much more accurate and achieve greater success if you reduce those global issues (tabletops) to the specific events (table legs) that cause them. Examples of specific events for the global issue of "I feel abandoned" could include:

The time my mother left me in the shopping mall when I was in second grade.

The time my father told me to leave home when I was twelve.

The time my third-grade teacher gave me that "I don't care about you" look.

These specific events are much easier to deal with than the global issues they created. If you deal with them one at a time without letting your attention shift, it will be easy to clear them—and by clearing the emotions stored in these small specific events, you can automatically repair the larger global issue.

To this point, I have provided more general examples like "fear of public speaking," "these nightmares," or "this anxiety." As a beginner, you can learn the process using general phrases like these, and your system will address the specifics behind the scenes. To be more direct and get more powerful results, however, it's better to break those general issues into the specific events that contribute to them.

For "these nightmares," simply take one nightmare at a time, or identify a difficult event that occurred around the time the nightmares began. For "fear of public speaking," make a list of all the events in which public speaking was uncomfortable for you and tap them away one by one. For issues like anxiety, stress, or depression, you are usually dealing with a combination of emotions so it may take a little longer to see significant results, but you can start by finding the past events that have upset you the most and address them with EFT.

For additional help in finding specific events to tap on, ask yourself questions like:

> *When did this problem start? What was I doing at the time? What was going on in my life?*
>
> *What does this issue remind me of?*

The Generalization Effect

That said, I want to acquaint you now with a fascinating feature of EFT. I call it the generalization effect because, after you address a few related problems with EFT, the process starts to generalize to all related problems. For example, someone who has a hundred traumatic memories of being abused usually finds that after using EFT and neutralizing only five or ten of them, they *all* vanish.

This is startling to some people because they have so many traumas in their life, they think they are in for unending sessions with these techniques. Not so—at least not usually. EFT often clears out a whole forest after cutting down just a few trees. You'll see an excellent example of this generalization effect in my session with Rich, the first veteran on the "Six Days at the V.A." video on www.EFTUniverse.com.

The Movie Technique and the Story Technique

When addressing specific events with EFT, we often use the Watch the Movie Technique or the Tell the Story Technique. In both methods, you review a past event while tapping to reduce its emotional charge. The difference between the two is that in the Movie Technique, you watch events unfold in your mind, as though you're watching a movie, whereas in the Story Technique, you describe the events aloud.

The "plot" of the movie or story is usually very short. If not, reduce the length down to one or two emotional crescendos because that sets up the target for EFT's aim. If jumping straight to the key event is too painful, however, the movie or story can begin a few minutes before the first emotional crescendo. The event may have hurt, but its retelling doesn't have to.

Unlike psychotherapy techniques that require clients to relive unpleasant past events in excruciating detail, EFT's approach is gentle and flexible. You watch the movie or tell the story until you reach a point that feels uncomfortable. Instead of forcing yourself to push on, just tap until the emotional intensity of that segment fades. When you feel comfortable again, resume the movie or story. When feelings rise again, tap until they subside. Eventually, you will be able to narrate the whole story without any emotional intensity and regain your freedom with respect to that memory.

Our bodies store traumas, and our mental movies are keys that unlock emotions stored with those traumas. Because EFT tapping reduces the emotional charge attached to past events, it transforms the traumas, memories, energy blocks, targeted body parts, and emotions that were previously locked together. With the emotional charge gone, the traumas become normal memories, the connections disappear, and the pain once associated with them vanishes as well.

EFT's Constricted Breathing Technique

The Constricted Breathing Technique is a breathing exercise enhanced by tapping which, despite its simplicity, offers numerous benefits. It is a popular demonstration in workshops and client sessions because most people have constricted breathing and it is eye-opening to experience the improvements that EFT generates in a minute or two. Increased oxygen levels are so important to health that practically everyone who tries this procedure feels better as a result. Daily use can help improve physical fitness, and because it's relaxing, the technique is an attitude-adjustment tool that can help you move from stressed or anxious to calm and serene in record time. This makes it an effective aid in improving performance as well as setting and reaching any new goal.

To use the technique, take two or three deep breaths. Take your time and don't hyperventilate. This step will stretch your lungs so that any EFT improvement in your breathing will not result from a normal "stretching effect."

Once you have stretched your lungs as far as they will go, take another deep breath. This time assess the deepness of your breath on a 0-to-10 scale, where 10 is your estimate of your maximum capacity. Most people start with numbers from 3 to 9. Those who rate their breath at a 10 (they are usually wrong) may find that, after EFT, they go to a 12 or 15.

Now do several rounds of EFT with Setup Phrases such as:

Even though my breathing is constricted, I deeply and completely accept myself.

Even though I can only fill my lungs to an 8…

Even though I'm not used to breathing deeply…

Be sure to include any physical or medical condition that could interfere, such as:

Even though I'm coming down with a cold [or have allergies or emphysema or a bruised rib] and it's hard to breathe, I deeply and completely accept myself.

After each round, take another deep breath and assess your 0-to-10 lung capacity. In the vast majority of cases, it keeps expanding and improving.

To clear any emotional cause of constricted or shallow breathing, ask yourself:

What does this constricted breath remind me of?

When have I felt constricted or smothered?

If there was an emotional reason for my constricted breath, what might it be?

Often these questions give big clues to important emotional issues. With the help of the Constricted Breathing Technique, whatever you feel upset, distressed, angry, disappointed, frustrated, guilty, irritated, sad, uncomfortable, or unhappy about can be more easily identified, incorporated into an EFT Setup Phrase, and tapped for.

Secondary Gain

Secondary gain is a psychiatric term meaning that the person has a reason for holding onto an undesirable condition, even though he or she may not recognize it.

The term applies to a wide variety of issues. An example would be a chronic pain case in which the patient will lose certain benefits by getting well, such as attention from others, monetary compensation for disability, or the ability to keep denying the original cause of the pain.

In metaphysics, the term "secondary gain" helps explain why we seem to run into barriers when it comes to manifesting our good. This occurs when we put a great deal of energy into visualizing, affirming, and treating for a new level of good and it either doesn't happen or the situation actually gets worse. The subconscious mind feels more secure in the disadvantaged state than in going for improvement. So while your conscious mind might be saying, *"I sincerely want to get over this problem,"* your subconscious screams, *"No, I don't!"*

If you suspect secondary gain, consider the following:

What benefits do you receive from your problem?

Does keeping the problem feel safe?

Does releasing it feel dangerous?

Does keeping the problem generate sympathy from others that you won't receive if you release the problem?

Does keeping the problem allow you to avoid unpleasant situations?

Does keeping the problem give you financial rewards that you won't receive without it?

Do you feel you don't deserve to get over the problem?

Do you fear that if you get better, something bad will happen?

Interestingly enough, secondary gain issues can be broken down into specific events, just like other issues. The process is more difficult because the problem is usually stated globally or generally, but if you keep asking yourself *"Why?"* or *"What's behind that?"* you are likely to find some specific events to address.

The Personal Peace Procedure

In my online tutorial on the EFT website, www.EFTUniverse.com, I describe the Personal Peace Procedure, which is an easy exercise that can help you tap away your issues one event at a time. This is especially helpful if you are having trouble finding your core issues or if you just want something to tap on every day. Although you may not be targeting the core issue behind a specific problem every time, you will be able to clear a large volume of unresolved emotions in a relatively short period of time. This is a different approach from targeting only the issues that contribute to specific problems, but the end result is often more complete.

Try it now. The sooner you start, the sooner you'll experience true personal peace.

1. **Make a list.** On a blank sheet of paper or at your computer, make a list of every bothersome specific event you can remember. If you don't find at least fifty, you are either going at this halfheartedly or you have been living on some other planet. Many people find hundreds.

2. **List everything.** While making your list you may find that some events don't seem to cause you any current discomfort. That's okay. List them anyway. The mere fact that you remember them suggests a need for resolution.

3. **Give each event a title** as though it is a mini-movie. Examples:

   Dad hit me in the kitchen.

   I stole Suzie's sandwich.

   I almost slipped and fell into the Grand Canyon.

   My third grade class ridiculed me when I gave that speech.

   Mom locked me in a closet for hours.

   Mrs. Adams told me I was stupid.

4. **Tap for the big ones.** When the list is complete, pick out the biggest redwoods in your negative forest (the ones closest to 10 on the 0-to-10 scale) and apply EFT to each one of them until you either laugh about it or just can't think about it anymore. Be sure to notice any aspects that come up and consider them separate trees in your negative forest. Apply EFT to them accordingly. Be sure to keep after each event until it

is resolved down to 0. After the biggest redwoods are removed, look for the next-biggest, and so on.

5. **Work on at least one movie per day**—preferably three—for three months. It takes only minutes per day. At this rate, you will resolve 90 to 270 specific events in three months. Then notice how your body feels better. Note, too, how your threshold for getting upset is much lower. Note how your relationships are better and how many of your therapy-type issues just don't seem to be there anymore. Revisit some specific events and notice how those previously intense incidents have faded into nothingness. Note any improvements in your life.

   I ask you to notice these things consciously because, unless you do, the quality healing you will undergo may be so subtle that you don't notice it. You may even dismiss it by saying, "Oh well, it was never much of a problem anyway." This happens repeatedly with EFT and thus I bring it to your awareness.

6. **If necessary, see your physician.** If you are taking prescription medications, you may feel the need to discontinue them. Please do so *only* under the supervision of a qualified health-care practitioner.

It is my hope that the Personal Peace Procedure will become a worldwide routine. A few minutes per day will make a monumental difference in school performance, the workplace, relationships, health, and our quality of life. But these are meaningless words unless you put the idea into practice. As my good friend Howard Wight says, "If you are ultimately going to do something important that will make a real difference...do it now."

Is EFT Working Yet?

Whenever EFT produces dramatic results, the changes are obvious. You start out afraid of heights and now you're comfortable leaning over a fire escape or climbing a ladder. You had a migraine headache and now you feel terrific. You were mad at your boss and now you're laughing.

But not every improvement occurs right away. Sometimes nothing seems to happen during your tapping session and you give up in disappointment, but then a few hours later or the following day, you notice that the problem has completely disappeared. EFT can have a delayed effect.

And not all improvements are obvious. Some occur so subtly that they are barely noticed or not noticed at all. Paying attention to all aspects of your life, not just the symptoms you are treating with EFT, will help you appreciate these subtle results.

In a case reported by EFT practitioner Chrissie Hardisty, a twenty-one-year-old client dropped out of college because of severe depression that did not respond to prescription antidepressants. Fortunately, it did respond to tapping and, as the client later reported, his lifelong spider phobia disappeared as well. Spiders didn't enter his mind during his tapping session, and he only noticed this profound change of attitude when his father called it to his attention. Instead of having a panic attack at the sight of a spider, he remained calm and relaxed.

June Campbell used EFT to help her friend Betty overcome her fear of flying. As a bonus, Betty's severe dental pain, which had not responded to painkillers, disappeared during the session. "Betty hadn't mentioned the pain so I hadn't addressed it during tapping," she says. "The stubborn dental pain was gone as if by magic. That was two days ago. The pain has not returned. Betty is not at all anxious about her upcoming flight, and she reports having a better night's sleep than she's had in quite some time."

EFT practitioner Margo Arrowsmith worked with a man who was afraid of banks. After tapping away this fear with EFT, he was not only able to go into and out of banks with ease, but his sinus congestion—which he hadn't mentioned or addressed—disappeared for the first time in years. She says, "I have worked with people for their feelings of guilt about some minor childhood incident, and their headaches disappeared. Talk to any EFT practitioners and they will tell you lots of stories of unexpected and delightful side effects."

How might EFT tapping affect you? Individual results vary, but EFT practitioners have seen many situations in which EFT corrects problems that were not addressed or even thought of during the tapping. These results include:

relief from insomnia   *lower stress levels*

improved digestion   *increasing patience*

fewer headaches   *a more relaxed attitude*

better overall health   *more energy*

improved range of motion *better relationships*

higher confidence levels   *faster healing from illness or injury*

increased efficiency   *improved memory*

growing optimism   *a reduction of fears and phobias*

relief from worry   *and more!*

Many of these changes can be overlooked if you aren't watching for them. Although there are many ways to keep track of the improvements that EFT produces, one of the simplest is to make a list of your life situations, your physical symptoms, and your feelings. Spend a few minutes each day or each week reviewing that list. Keeping a journal, diary, or notebook will help you remember details that might otherwise go unnoticed. Pay attention to the observations of others, too. They are evidence of transformations taking place within you.

This inventory is especially important if it seems as though EFT is not working. If you can't seem to release your emotional intensity, you still have an out-of-control craving, your elbow still hurts, you still feel depressed, or whatever you're addressing won't seem to budge, consider the possibility that other improvements are contributing to your success with the original problem.

In EFT, results can come quickly, or they can involve the repeated tapping sessions that we call "peeling the onion." You clear up one aspect of a problem only to have another appear, and it isn't until several of these layered aspects are dealt with that the problem completely goes away.

If it seems as though nothing is happening, don't give up. You might feel just as sad and discouraged as you did last week, but you may be sleeping better, or other drivers on the road don't annoy you the way they usually do. Your elbow may be as sore as it was yesterday, but you're criticizing your kids less and enjoying them more, or friends notice that you seem more relaxed. You're still helpless to resist chocolate ice cream, but you feel more energetic and complete a project at work ahead of schedule. Any of these or a thousand other small improvements suggests that your EFT tapping is producing deep-level changes.

Upcoming Examples

I have already described EFT as a flexible healing tool and, as you can see in my book *The EFT Manual* or in my DVDs available on the EFT website, not all EFT sessions follow the basic instruction exactly.

This book includes an extensive collection of real stories about people who have used EFT for themselves or a friend, relative, client, or student for back pain. These examples will help you understand how to use EFT in different situations, and how the basic principles you already know can be applied to an actual case—like yours.

I will provide plenty of narrative as we go so that you can see where the basic principles are being illustrated and where people have used their own variation to address a unique situation. Emotional issues are often complex, and there are many different ways to be specific or thorough with EFT. Accordingly, some people use fairly global or general approaches and others get all the way down to specific events, but they are all peeling away layers as they go.

One of the most obvious variations will be the extended Setup Phrases. With experience, you may find that using a longer description in the Setup to target your issue produces better results. By being more creative in the Setup, you might trigger more memories than with the default or standard Setup, and that can help you get to deeper core issues.

One common misconception, however, is that the "right words" in the Setup are the magical key to results with EFT. This is not the case, although the examples you see in this book might leave you with that impression.

If you find that you "don't know what to say" in your Setup, you can always use the default or standard Setup Phrase, which is:

> *Even though I have this _____, I deeply and completely accept myself.*

If you can't find a word for the _____, or if you aren't getting results, your Setup is probably too global, vague, or general, and you need to look deeper for a specific event related to the problem.

Once you find a specific event, use the Setup to describe it the same way you would tell it to a friend, and use the Tell the Story Technique to tap away the intensity one crescendo at a time. If addressing that event doesn't do the trick, then look for similar events, or try the Personal Peace Procedure.

Remember, getting results with EFT is more about *"What are you tapping for?"* than *"What words are you saying?"*

I encourage you to consider EFT a universal healing tool, something that can improve any and every part of your life. The more often you use it, the more likely you are to experience benefits in not just one or two areas but in all aspects of your being—and the more likely you are to resolve the original problem completely.

2

Tapping Away Cravings

Using EFT to reduce cravings is a very common first step when addressing weight-loss issues. While this approach does not initially target specific events, you can be very specific with the decription of your cravings, and you may find that cravings are often metaphors for under-lying issues. The bigger payoff is that when you have a craving, your underlying food issues are triggered and looking for attention. This is the best time to use EFT on anything—when the intensity is high.

A craving is a strong desire, an intense longing, for a special something. It can be for anything, even raw car-rots, but among those who would like to lose weight, raw carrot cravings are rare. Ice cream, chocolate, macaroni and cheese, pound cake, cookies, and other filling, satisfy-ing, high-fat, high-carb treats are the comfort foods that keep calling.

Those who are new to EFT have trouble believing that tapping on acupuncture points can interrupt, diminish, or even destroy a craving, but it happens all the time. I've received many reports from EFT professionals who distribute potato chips, candy, and other highly craved snacks in EFT weight-loss workshops. At first people fight over the items, saying things like, "It's a 10 and I'll kill you for it!!" But as they tap while saying,

> *Even though I have this incredible craving for _____, I deeply and completely accept myself...*

they are startled to realize that the craving has completely disappeared. It can happen in just a minute or two.

If the simple Setup above doesn't do the trick, enhancing the description usually will. Try smelling the item, tasting just a little, holding it in you hand, or doing anything else that might help you discover apsects of your craving that haven't been addressed yet, and incorporate these observations into your Setup. For example:

> *Even though that chocolate is making my mouth water and I can't even look at it without drooling, I deeply and completely accept myself.*

> *Even though I really want those potato chips, and I can already smell how fresh and crispy they would be if I were to open that bag, I deeply and completely accept myself.*

Once their cravings have been "tapped away," it is often difficult for people to taste, touch, or even look at the very same foods they were excited about moments before. Someone who loves potato chips will frown and say, "The whole package smells rancid." A chocolate lover will complain that a fresh, expensive piece tastes weird or waxy.

EFT Research and Weight Loss

The evidence supporting EFT's effectiveness for cravings isn't just anecdotal. A 2009 study conducted at Griffith University in Australia by psychologists Peta Stapleton, PhD, and Terri Sheldon examined the effectiveness of EFT for food cravings. The active treatment group consisted of 96 overweight or obese adults who received EFT, while a control group of 47 overweight or obese adults received no treatment. The treatment group received two hours of EFT per week for four weeks. Weight, food cravings, the perceived power of food, restraint capabilities, and psychological symptoms like anxiety and depression were assessed before and after the four weeks of EFT as well as six months later. Data analysis showed that EFT resulted in statistically significant improvements on every scale except restraint, with even restraint showing improvement at the six-month mark. EFT successfully controlled the food cravings of this group, and it continued to help study subjects control their cravings—and their weight—even six months later.

In a separate study, Dawson Church of Soul Medicine Institute gathered data from 216 participants who took one-day EFT courses at five professional conferences. Most of the participants were healthcare workers such as doctors, nurses, psychotherapists, chiropractors, and alternative medicine practitioners. They all had high stress levels when coming into the workshop, but the severity of their psychological symptoms decreased by 45 percent afterwards. Those results were highly statistically significant ($p < .001$).

What was interesting from a weight-loss perspective was that participants were asked to rate their cravings on the 0-to-10 scale for substances such as chocolate, alcohol, sweets, cake, tobacco, or drugs. After just 20 minutes of EFT, their cravings dropped by 83 percent! These results were also highly statistically significant (p < .001).

Audrey Brooks, PhD, a psychologist at the University of Arizona at Tucson, measured the cravings of people taking two-day EFT workshops taught by a variety of EFT practitioners. She too found highly statistically significant drops in cravings as well as improvements in psychological problems like anxiety and depression. And when she re-measured the participants' psychological issues three months later, they were still better than when they walked into the workshop.

To appreciate how quickly and effectively EFT can work for your own issues, including weight loss and uncontrollable cravings, consider the following reports.

Linda Compton started a "Roots of Weight" class and used EFT to help with the many addictive substances that contribute to being overweight. I think you will find her message filled with evidence about how EFT works in this area. Some people seemingly get completely over their cravings rapidly while others have increased cravings for something else.

Intense Cravings in a Weight-loss Class

by Linda Compton

At one point, I started a class for women called the Roots of Weight. There were ten women in the class and we met every Thursday from 7 to 9 p.m.

At the third class I taught EFT and the women tapped for everything from chips to cigarettes, Milano cookies, StarBucks peanut butter cookies, wine, and vodka.

One woman said she had the unusual habit of chewing eight packs of gum every night. She would fall asleep chewing gum, wake up two hours later, and eat a one-pound pack of raisins. Then she would chew more gum and fall asleep. The gum had to come from a particular store and it had to be Doublemint in the green wrapper and Spearmint in the white wrapper. She would repeat this cycle every night.

She told me, "I have a master's degree in psychology. I should be able to stop this, but I feel out of control."

She tapped for the raisins only and ten days later, she still doesn't want them. She told me she looked at the raisins on the shelf and thought, "Oh, there are those raisins." She had no desire to eat the raisins. She didn't crave them any more at all. And although she was happy about the raisins, she said the intensity of the craving for the gum increased. Next, she tapped for the gum chewing. She called a few days later to say that she had not had any gum, nor did she want any. She had four packs in her drawer and had absolutely no craving for it.

I spoke with her shortly thereafter and she said this is a miracle. She has been doing this behavior of chewing gum and eating raisins all night for two years. She made numerous visits to the doctor and was told not to worry about it, that it would soon pass. She even brought up the idea that she might have a nutritional deficiency, like a lack of chromium, but the doctor told her the research wasn't in on that. She is ecstatic.

She is not the only one in the class who stopped cravings. Another woman eats five small donuts a day. She is down to one and a half. Another ate three bags of corn nuts last Wednesday and is addicted to potato chips, pork rinds, and anything salty. She told me she hasn't had any of those items since she tapped for her cravings.

I tapped for sugar with the class and haven't had any since. I have also let go of coffee, popcorn, and ice cream. And although we could be tapping for all these food items at one time, I know that particular cravings are motivated by particular emotions and sometimes physical conditions.

One friend let go of the grief she had been feeling for her deceased mother. There were songs she could not stand to listen to and is now OK with. Another client let go of coffee and her fear of selling real estate. She now is working full time selling real estate and teases me about "f-ing up her coffee thing."

In my Roots of Weight class, these women are exploring the deep roots of their beliefs so that they can see clearly how the beliefs branch out to undesired behaviors, creating undesired results, such as undesired weight. One of the women found this so profound that she downloaded the EFT manual to study.

This is so wonderful. The woman with the gum-chewing habit demonstrates how large this whole energy psychology is. She just can't believe she only had to tap once to heal it.

❖ ❖ ❖

Whether it is chocolate, popcorn, or a special snack or dessert, our systems can develop a major case of the Yum-Yums and cause us to overeat many things. Collette Streicher's client faced this dilemma with regard to peanuts and used EFT to effectively diminish her cravings.

Notice how Colette's client started with a craving, peeled away emotional layers, and uncovered a supporting emotional issue. It's the underlying issues we really want to address, so whenever you're tapping, be on the lookout for them.

Overcoming a Food Craving
by Collette Streicher and Chris

My client, Chris, sent me this great letter about how she eliminated a peanut craving with all the details and some humor, too. She hopes it can help others.

Dear Colette,

I am writing this note to tell you how much the EFT has been helping me with food cravings. What I absolutely love about working with this tool is the flexibility and availability of using my fingertips to conquer problems that used to overwhelm me.

I have long struggled with food issues. I know I have a lot of great reasons to lose weight, but I could never get past the thought that I would have to let go of food that I really loved, especially peanuts. If I were ever stranded on a desert island, it would be a long, long time before I starved because you can bet I would have a huge pack of peanuts in my purse, one in a certain pocket of my briefcase, and if I had driven to that island, there would be a jar or two rolling around on the car's floorboard. So, as I've learned, from you and others on the EFT website, I started with whatever feeling came up first.

Even though I really can't stand the idea of giving up peanuts, I deeply and completely accept myself.

Even though I'm angry that I am forced to give up peanuts…

Forced? Who was forcing me? I couldn't think of anyone standing between peanuts and me. So I went with that.

Even though I don't know who is forcing me to stop eating peanuts…

Even though it is me who is being so forceful…

Even though I feel forceful when I am eating peanuts...

Now this rang true for me. I have always known that part of the appeal of nuts for me is the physical crunching and chewing. I guess I feel like I am getting somewhere by doing all that chewing.

Even though chewing and crunching feels forceful...

Then as I was tapping the above statement, it came to me. I used to get angry at my ex-husband, the one who was constantly nagging me about losing weight.

Even though my ex tried to force me to lose weight, I ate anyway, 'cause nobody can stop me if I don't want to stop.

Even though I can't say anything about not wanting to lose weight, I can chew and chew these peanuts forcefully.

Then I really got it that the act of chewing was about biting back my feelings and biting back my words. I could feel the anger in my jaws! By this time I was just tapping on the points with these Reminder Phrases:

This biting back my feelings.

This biting back my words.

These angry jaws.

These forceful jaws.

Then I felt sad because that was the only way I could express myself in that situation, so again, I tapped on:

> *This sadness.*
> *This peanut sadness.*
> *This chewing sadness.*
> *This feeling alone.*

Then I felt better, so I stopped. Most of the anger was gone. I didn't test myself, because I was a little melancholy that I had to do all this work around peanuts and chewing. I could have tapped on the shame of having this issue in the first place, but I didn't. I know if I had been in a session with you, we might have gone deeper, but I felt satisfied at the time. In fact, I didn't really think to see if peanuts still had a charge with me. I started doing something else.

The oddest thing (though maybe not to you) was that I didn't even think about peanuts again until I was in line at the bank and I saw the emergency package I kept in my purse. I hadn't eaten peanuts in days! Then it became weeks. I can truthfully say I am not peanutty anymore!

Notice Chris's references to anger, sadness, shame, and feeling alone. These are all aspects of the issue with her ex-husband. If the peanut craving came back after this session, or if the overall food issue persisted, I might look deeper into the specific events with her ex-husband, or see if there is something similar in childhood to address.

❀ ❀ ❀

Alyson Raworth's client in Scotland had a major chocolate craving. Notice how she amplifies the "yummi-ness" and appeal of the chocolate to truly tune her client into the craving. Nestlé's Yorkies, which are popular in the U.K., are marketed as a man's chocolate bar. In this session, Alyson has her client massage his Sore Spot on the upper chest instead of tapping the Karate Chop point while reciting his Setup Phrase. The two can be used interchangeably. For more about the Sore Spot, see Appendix A.

Hitting a Chocolate Craving Head-on

by Alyson Raworth

I have been doing sessions with a male client who desperately wanted to lose weight but who had a chocolate fixation. He tried and tried but although he seemed to have willpower, he didn't have enough for this chocolate thing.

As the rest of his diet was sensible, I concentrated on the chocolate. I put some pieces of Yorkie on the table in front of him. His level of desire was above a 10.

I started with having him massage his Sore Spot while saying:

Even though my chocolate thing is intense, I love my body. Although I really love and want that yummy Yorkie, I love and respect my body.

His level went down to 9.

Then I did a big one:

> *Even though I can taste the texture of that gorgeous velvety sweetness which is just so yummy that my tongue is swirling round in my mouth in anticipation of popping that piece in front of me into my mouth, I love and respect myself and choose to have the imagination to see myself slim.*

He looked strangely at me and had one of those sighs. He said that he had never been able to imagine himself actually slim!

The wording was then changed to:

> *Even though I am just an old tub of lard, not good for anything, not even good for getting slim, I do love and respect my body and mind.*

He laughed and laughed at that and said that the chocolate looked different now. I asked him to explain and he said that it had somehow lost its appeal!

That was the turning point. I asked him how much he wanted to eat the chocolate now and he said that he didn't want it at all. His level was a complete zero! Brilliant!

We are going to work on his self-image next and build up confidence and self-esteem.

❊ ❊ ❊

You may have noticed the use of "I love and respect my body" in the preceding report's Setup Phrases. That statement is a cousin to "I deeply and completely accept myself" because it adds an element of self-acceptance to the Setup.

You may have also noticed "I choose to have the imagination to see myself slim." This is an EFT variation that uses affirmations to trigger new aspects. Obviously, Alyson was savvy enough to know that an overall self-image issue might have been a bigger contributor to the craving than the Yorkie. By using the affirmation, she was able to test the waters and found a valuable direction for her next round of tapping.

If a craving doesn't disappear in record time, it is probably attached to an emotional issue that needs to be addressed before the craving can be diminished. Sergio Lizarraga from Mexico illustrates this next with a brief report.

Chocolate Cravings and Childhood Poverty
by Sergio Lizarraga

A friend was struggling with her weight issues. I introduced her to a basic routine of EFT to help eliminate her chocolate cravings, which were the major contributor to her overweight problem. But when she tapped for her chocolate cravings directly, it did not help at all. When we talked about it later on, she told me about her childhood in poverty and how she could not have candies or chocolates then. Now that she is an adult she wants the chocolates she could not have as a child. I suggested tapping on:

Even though I could not have chocolate when I was a child, I deeply and completely accept myself.

Even though I wanted a chocolate when I was a child...

Three weeks later she contacted me again, very happy. She says that by doing the tapping in this way her craving totally disappeared. Now she is losing weight and feeling much better. Needless to say she is using EFT for a lot of issues in her life and for her family as well.

Something interesting to mention here is that I have never met my friend in person. We got in touch through a Spanish EFT webpage that I own. All the conversations and ideas shared have been done through instant messages and emails!

✷ ✷ ✷

In the preceding case, Sergio was able to find some underlying emotional issues connected to the craving and apparently didn't have to go any further. When using EFT for your own craving, if you have tapped on similar issues and still aren't seeing results, you could be more specific by working with the events themselves, like "the time when my father wouldn't let me have chocolate..." and any others that cause intensity. Once all the related memories have lost their "grip," that part of the issue is likely to be released for good.

In this next article by Dr. Shelley Malka, you will see how she helped her client get to the true emotional issues behind cravings that just wouldn't go away. Notice how the tapping process and Shelley's gentle suggestions along the way reduced a frustrating craving down to what seems to be a specific event. Also note how Shelley was able to address the event even though she didn't know any of the details. This case illustrates why it is often important to seek the help of an experienced professional for best results.

What was *Really* Behind Those Cravings?
by Dr. Shelley Malka

The following story demonstrates clearly that any craving or addiction is not about the object we crave at all. Rather, the craved object is a substitute for anxiety that lies beneath the addiction. Once we access that disallowed or forbidden feeling, the craving disappears as if by magic. And you as the therapist or helper don't have to know what's really going on for this process to work wonders.

Odette was a client I knew well. She called me over the phone one day asking me to please help her work through her craving for chocolate and cake that had been with her the last few days. Intensity for these foods was building and she knew she couldn't hold out much longer on her own without blowing her diet. She had tapped consistently but couldn't get to whatever it was that was clearly holding up her craving.

"What triggered this?" I asked. "You've been much better with chocolate and cake recently."

"I know I have," she said. "That's why I'm so frustrated. I just can't work this one out and the craving is ballooning."

"OK," I said. "Just go to the Karate Chop point and let's start."

Even though I don't know what triggered this… I was doing fine…doing much better…and then the last few days I haven't been able to get cake out of my mind…and chocolate…I don't know why…

Nothing emerged and, looking for a door to go in, I asked if she had a craving right then. She said, "No, not right now, but I know that if I wasn't on the phone to you, I'd head straight for the chocolate."

"You don't have the craving now perhaps because I'm here and you feel safe." I let her tap on this awareness a bit. "When did you have this craving? Could you allow your inner mind to go to where you were, what was happening when you first noticed this feeling of needing cake?" Tap, tap.

"Well I think the first time I started this cake-feeling I was in the car. If there'd been a place to buy chocolate, I think I would have stopped right there."

"Go into that moment," I suggested "Just be in the car and allow that feeling to surface…I'm in the car…just tap around the points in the car and all of a sudden I want cake…all of a sudden I'm looking around for somewhere to buy chocolate." Her level of intensity was between 5 and 6 on a scale of 0 to 10.

Even though I'm a 5 or 6 right now…And I don't know what it is…Even though it's intensifying, that's good, that's why I phoned you, to find out what this is…

At that moment, she burst out crying. "I think I do know," she said. "I can't believe it's this...I had no idea. I can't believe it's this...but that's what's coming up."

We tapped a few rounds on "this awareness... this realization." Then she said, "And it's a lose-lose situation!" I immediately referred her back to the Karate Chop point.

Even though it's a lose-lose situation...

Even though no matter what I do, I'll lose out...

We did quite a bit of this. I didn't add anything. I wanted whatever needed to surface, to just float up to consciousness. We tapped on the feelings that arose.

Even though I'm scared...

Whenever there's a fear we're afraid to face—fear of the fear as it's often called—we're usually holding an underlying belief that if we know what that fear is, we won't be able to cope with it. So I threw this in:

Even though I'm scared, and I don't know if I can handle it...And that's making me crave chocolate and cake...

"That's right!" she exclaimed. "I don't!" More sobs. I backtracked here so she could process the steps and integrate the parts as we traveled round and round the points:

It's a lose-lose situation and I'm scared because I don't know if I can handle it...no matter what I do, I'll lose and I don't know if I can handle that...it's mak-

ing me crave chocolate and cake because I'm so anxious about this lose-lose…I want to stuff it down with chocolate and cake.

"Anything!" she cried. "Even chicken and potatoes!" Well, this was a new aspect she hadn't realized before, so I took her back to the Karate Chop point:

Even though this lose-lose is making me crave anything, even chicken and potatoes, and it's all to keep my anxiety down…

This anxiety that I can't handle the lose-lose…this anxiety that I can't handle my feelings about this lose-lose…calming this anxiety with any food so that I can obsess about food and my weight rather than deal with this lose-lose anxiety.

"Yeah," she agreed, "that's what I do, all right." But she was definitely calmer, having found the issue underpinning her craving.

We checked her craving. She was still a 4 or 5 on the 0-to-10 scale, even though she had stopped crying. "It's because I haven't found the core yet," she said. "And I'm anxious about not finding it."

We did a whole lot more tapping on this—to calm her, to make her anxiety OK, to challenge the assumptions in her unconscious mind that she couldn't handle the lose-lose (whatever that was, since I had no clue). I asked what the craving was like and she said it was still 4 or 5 out of 10 "because I don't know how he'll take it." Here was another aspect that slipped out, so seemingly innocuous as to have us believe she'd known about it all along.

Even though I don't know how he'll take it...

Her tears and sobs started up again.

Even though I have no idea how he'll take it and that's the real concern, the real anxiety...up to now I haven't allowed myself to know how anxious I am about that...I was scared I wouldn't be able to handle it...I truly was scared to know this because it seemed too big for me...

By now her voice was softer and more pliable. Things had changed. So we checked her craving again. "It's much better!" she said. "I don't need the chocolate anymore!"

I asked her to do what she could to get that craving back either for chocolate, or cake or chicken and potatoes or anything I got her to make the images bigger and brighter and smell the chocolate in her mind... but the craving was gone. Furthermore, Odette not only knew she could now handle her feelings about how he'd take it but it was also no longer lose-lose. She had found a solution to make it easy.

I said, "So now that you know what IT is, you can tap for that, without me, and you no longer have to eat yourself into oblivion." She laughed again. "I feel such relief. It always amazes me how it's never about the cake or the chocolate, is it?" I said goodbye to Odette and looked at my watch. The entire session had taken approximately 15 minutes. And I never did find out what "it" was.

❊ ❊ ❊

EFT usually gets rid of immediate cravings in short order. When that doesn't happen, there is almost always a deeper issue behind the craving. Such was the case in this article by Ilana Weiler from Israel. Note how important memories showed up during the EFT process, pointing the way to the problem's core issue.

A Craving Vanishes for a Skeptical Doctor

by Ilana Weiler

Recently I attended a birthday party and had the pleasure of meeting a group of amazing women. I assume we all know that scenario where we find ourselves in a social gathering and sooner or later the subject of EFT is brought up. One of the women said, "What is this EFT? Is it this stupid thing where one taps on himself looking like a monkey?"

Well, that's a chance to catch the ball. She is a highly positioned doctor but, nonetheless, I asked her if she would like to try it. To my great surprise, she agreed. I am writing all the details of this event to encourage you, the reader who doesn't yet feel confident with EFT, to not only Try It on Everything but also Try It on Everybody—anytime.

So this woman (I will call her Lea), wanted to try EFT for her uncontrollable desire for sweets. I asked her what on the table she wanted to eat the most. She said she wanted everything, but mostly the cake. On the scale of 0 to 10 she wanted it at a level of 8. I asked her what it was about that cake that she wanted so much. She said it was the sweetness of it.

Even though I want that sweet cake so much…

We used the words sweet, sweet cake, and sweetness as Reminder Phrases.

After one round Lea said, "I am like an elephant that grabs everything sweet with its trunk. I am like a vacuum cleaner."

After a few rounds I handed her the piece of cake. Now it had a level of intensity of 6 out of 10. We kept tapping while she suddenly said, "Oh, I have a flashback of a memory when I was about three years old. My father used to buy me those sugar candies that looked like crystals."

I kept tapping on her as she talked, astonished by the fact she had recalled a memory she had never remembered in 50 years. And then came another. She said, "I remember we used to go to the zoo, and my father always had these little bags filled with sweets. And now I remember how he used to feed me patiently this sweet porridge."

She was absolutely a pleasure to work with, so freely cooperating with the process of EFT. I was very touched by this gush of memories and she was, too. I asked Lea if she missed her father and she said she missed him terribly. Bingo.

Even though I miss my father terribly…physically and emotionally I miss my father…I miss him so much.

Even though I miss my sweet father, I miss our sweet relationship, I miss all those sweet memories, I accept my feelings and respect myself.

For Reminder Phrases, we used *my sweet father… our sweet relationship…my sweet memories.*

She said she understood that this craving for sugar was a substitute for her relationship with her father. I continually tapped on her as she suddenly said she could see herself as an adolescent, wearing a medallion of the peace symbol. "I want to make peace within me," she said.

After tapping for that I gave her the piece of cake and she repelled it with her whole body. "I can't even think of putting it in my mouth!" It was an amazing demonstration of getting to the core issue quickly. The whole thing took about 20 minutes. What a sweet process!

❀ ❀ ❀

In the next report, Dorothy Goudie from New Zealand gives us a classic example of how EFT neutralized a craving for ice cream. Notice the specific language she and her client used to describe the craving. If you just try to describe your craving the way you would to a good friend, this is the kind of language you might use. These detailed descriptions in the Setup help trigger the intensity more completely, and they assist the tapping process in correcting the related disruptions.

EFT for Ice Cream Cravings

by Dorothy Goudie

A woman with a weight problem narrowed her cravings down to several items with one being over-indulgence in ice cream—especially the ones coated in chocolate.

In New Zealand we have a chocolate-coated ice cream on a stick called a Topsy. This was her favorite. As we talked about the Topsy, she rated her craving at an intensity level of 10 out of 10. When I produced one and started to peel the wrapper off, she was salivating. By the time I put it in her hand and asked her just to smell it, her craving was way over a 10.

We put the ice cream to one side, away from her but where she could see it. While tapping on her Karate Chop point, I started by saying, *"I just love those Topsys."*

"Oh!" she exclaimed, "I can smell that beautiful sweet smell on your fingers." At this point she took over with the words pouring out, so I just repeated back to her what she was saying and continuously tapped while she was doing this.

The smell in particular is divine, and the creamy feel of the chocolate with the cool ice cream just melts in your mouth and flows over your tongue.

I just love ice cream, it is sooo good, and I can't get enough of it.

Love the taste, love the smell, just love everything about ice cream.

Surely ice cream can't be that fattening.

Oh I know it is but I just can't resist, love that cool feel in the mouth.

Love that smell, it's so sweet.

Delicious, makes me feel so good.

We did six or seven rounds of tapping on this and then took a pause while I asked how she was feeling now about ice cream. She had a blank look on her face, quite startled. It was almost as though it took a moment or two to realize that her previous thoughts were no longer so.

I suggested that she take another smell of the Topsy and give me a rating on the 0-to-10 scale. She took the ice cream and sniffed, and sniffed again, and with shock on her face said, "I can't smell anything. It's like plastic. My nose must be blocked. Did you switch the ice cream? You couldn't have done that, I was watching. I don't want to eat that. There is no pleasure in something that smells like plastic."

I suggested that she might like to take a bite of it and test it but she refused, saying that she couldn't bear to eat something that smelled like that.

An hour later, as she was ready to leave, we tested again with the same results. The intensity of her craving was still at a zero. She could not believe that her lifetime passion for ice cream could vanish in ten minutes.

I then asked her to take the Topsy and throw it in the rubbish. She took the ice cream in her hand and just stopped, shock showing in her face and body. She said, "I can't throw this away, what a waste, you could wrap it and someone else could eat it. You can't waste money on food like that and just throw it away."

Wow! Here we had another aspect. I walked her to the rubbish bin and said, "Now throw it in." She did but was visibly shaken. Back we went to tapping again on this new aspect. We tapped on all of the above that she had said, plus much more came up and I just tapped as she spoke.

If food is in front of you then you must eat it all. You can't have any waste. Clean your plate. Food costs money and you can't waste it. You'll be punished if you waste it. You're being greedy if you take food and don't eat it.

After several minutes and many rounds and much emotion, she calmed down. Although I didn't check her intensity initially, it was obviously 10 out of 10 and now it was down to zero. She went to the rubbish bin, looked at the ice cream, which was now melting, and said, "You'll have a nice sticky mess in there." No more emotion over waste.

She now has a tool to handle her addiction. I am in awe at the stunning simplicity of this EFT procedure.

* * *

A very important element of the above session is when Dorothy asked the client to throw the Topsy away.

This produced a new aspect to address with EFT, and I call that "testing the results." As I have mentioned before, when there are aspects of the issue left unaddressed, the issue will tend to come back. Whenever it seems as though the intensity is gone, find creative ways to verify that information and you will often find there is more to do.

Using EFT to address cravings directly is a great first step toward changing how you respond to food. In most cases, you can see immediate results and it is easy to see how EFT is helping you achieve your goals. However, even after EFT has been successful in eliminating one craving, or even a few cravings, any related emotional issues that have not been addressed can cause those cravings to come back in time.

For that reason, I encourage you to continue learning how to dig deeper and find the core issues behind your challenges with weight loss.

Food Addictions

Food addictions are like cravings, only more so.

In my experience, addictions that are primarily physical can be broken quite readily with EFT. The emotional ones take more time, care, and skill because the real problem isn't a simple physical craving. It is the need to tranquilize some strong unresolved emotions—*and until those emotions are resolved*, the addict will continue with the existing addiction or switch to another one.

I've worked with my share of people who no longer want their coffee, chocolate, or alcohol after one or two rounds of EFT. I've also had my share of people with seemingly endless emotional issues who truly *needed* their addictive substances or behaviors until an emotional clearing of their negative jungle occurred. It was their best solution to the problem until the causes could be eliminated. This can take time, of course.

You may notice that the cases in this chapter illustrate not only deeper emotional issues, but a higher level of experience with EFT as well. Most of these stories were submitted by experienced EFT practitioners and/or licensed therapists who have a more complete understanding of emotional issues and how to navigate through them.

I include these examples so you can see how deep the emotional issues can run, and how an experienced EFT professional might find and address them.

Improving your EFT skills will require good detective work to lead you to the specific issues that need attention, and good testing methods will let you know when there is more work to be done. You will see some great examples of both in this chapter, so feel free to try any of these approaches on your own issues.

In the first report, John Digby from the U.K. alertly uses EFT for physical symptoms that "show up" as he helps his client with a chocolate addiction.

It is always interesting to see how emotions show up as physical symptoms. People sweat when they're nervous, get a headache when they are stressed, or feel a knot in their stomach when they're scared. In this case, you will see that once the physical craving was tapped away, the emotions were still there and showed up in several physical forms.

When working on your own cravings or addictions, pay close attention to changes in your body, and be sure to address them with EFT. Because they represent aspects of the issue you are trying to resolve, they can lead you to deeper issues. Remember that even if you start by tapping on something global or general, emotional layers will be peeled away, revealing unexpected memories and very important clues for your healing process.

EFT for a Chocolate Addiction Triggers Symptoms
by John Digby

I run my practice from an office in a multi-use block of start-up companies and am opposite the kitchen, where I bump into most of the other occupants from time to time. One of the ladies that I speak with runs a local Weight Watchers group and had vouchsafed to me that she had a real addiction to *chocolate!* Now there's a surprise! Last Thursday I met her in the kitchen and this time asked her if she could spare ten minutes to see if I could help. She said OK.

We sat down and I showed her a small packet of German chocolate that I keep for demonstration purposes when running workshops. Her level of intensity was 9.5 on the 0-to-10 scale. I asked her to tap the Karate Chop point while she smelled the chocolate and described it to me. We then went onto EFT's Basic Recipe using reminder words like *smooth, yummy, warm, comforting, dribbling,* and *I really want it.* We breathed deeply and sighed. I asked for her level of intensity and she said there was none but that she felt sick.

We then did one shortcut round on feeling sick in the pit of her stomach and I asked for her level of intensity again. At this point she said she no longer felt sick but had a headache over her left eyebrow. After another short version for "sharp pain over my left eye," I asked her level of intensity again. Now she was completely clear and willing to throw the chocolate in the waste bin.

I found the diverse aspects of this five-minute session very interesting and was bowled over today when she looked in to say a heartfelt thanks. She said that since our session, she was feeling a lot more grounded and alert to the world and life in general. She really does seem a new woman, and all in five minutes. She has booked her place on my next introductory EFT workshop, and we are both looking forward to it immensely.

❋ ❋ ❋

In this next report, Dr. Carol Solomon describes a weight-related tapping session that reveals some emotional themes common among people with weight problems, like a need for approval or a need for attention. Dr. Solomon has previous experience with cases of this kind, and she is able to suggest directions for the session that beginners may not be able to replicate on their own. However, if any of these directions feel as though they fit for you, do a few similar rounds of tapping and see where they take you.

This case also illustrates more global uses of EFT, as seen in the various Setup Phrases. Global language is generally more effective if you use it with a longer term plan, and as you will see, this client tapped every day for a month and was encouraged to use EFT as a daily practice.

For faster results, this client's past issues could be broken down into specific events and the sting from these events could be "tapped away" quickly.

You will also see new aspects showing up as physical symptoms, just as we saw in the previous case. An interesting twist here is that Dr. Solomon treats them as metaphors for her client's emotional issues by suggesting that her client's family is a "pain in the neck" and that they give her a backache.

Morbidly Obese Woman Stops Feeling Hungry
by Dr. Carol Solomon

My client Jean was morbidly obese and had been unable to lose weight for many years. No matter what she tried, it would only last a short time before her eating got out of control again. Like many clients with persistent food and weight issues, Jean was holding onto old childhood hurts. She felt deprived as a child. Her mother was emotionally needy, and her sister, "the beautiful one," got most of the attention. Jean only got attention for being "responsible."

What Jean didn't get from her family, she gave to herself. Jean didn't think that she could get love and attention from her family, so she "settled" for food.

It didn't stop her from continuing to try to get her family's approval, even as an adult. Jean spent her entire life in search of the love and attention she didn't get from her family while hating herself for not being the one they gave it to. Jean's low self-esteem led to excessive pleasing behavior, in which she hid her true self while being unable to set limits. I don't know anything that will create stress more quickly than saying "yes" to everything!

Hanging onto her excess weight became a symbol for the only kind of attention Jean thought she could get. These patterns became obvious in one of my EFT sessions with her.

Even though I need to be needed…

Even though I need to show them how responsible I am…

She added:

Even though my fat gives me negative attention, and otherwise they ignore me, I love and accept myself anyway.

Even though I've spent my whole life breaking my back trying to please them.

At this point, Jean said her back started to hurt.

Even though they give me a backache…

Then the pain moved to her neck.

Even though they are a big pain in the neck, I love and accept myself completely.

Even though I can't accept that I'm not going to get the attention I want from them, I love and accept myself completely.

Even though I can't say no because they might think I'm not responsible, and that's all I have…

Even though I need to hang onto this fat to get attention, otherwise I'm invisible, I love and accept myself anyway.

Even though I'm still trying to prove myself, I approve of myself and I accept where I am in this process.

Jean's back and neck pain disappeared immediately. She tapped for a few minutes per day for about a month using a combination of these statements. I encouraged her to make EFT a daily practice. She is now steadily losing one to two pounds per week and she has stopped feeling "hungry" all the time. As a bonus, she no longer feels that she needs to say "yes" to every request and is feeling much happier.

❊ ❊ ❊

Although it seems like a nice little bonus, the change in Jean's overall behavior is one of the most powerful, yet subtle, benefits of using EFT. In many cases, we address pain, or weight loss, or some other current complaint, but by cleaning up the unresolved emotional events behind them, major shifts can happen. Eventually, the past is no longer unresolved or painful, and all of our conditioned behaviors, beliefs, and habits that we adopted in the past are no longer necessary. That's what we call emotional freedom!

The following report by Tam Llewellyn of the U.K. provides clear evidence of the link between addictions and unresolved emotional issues. His client could drink alcohol socially with no signs whatsoever of alcoholism.

However, when she drank a specific brand of beer—Budweiser—her drinking of *that* beer became uncontrollable.

Much of the "comfort" we derive from "comfort foods" has similar links to the past, and putting your EFT detective skills to use in finding them may help control your appetite just as dramatically as Tam's client controlled her appetite for Budweiser.

This session begins with a very simple application of basic EFT and demonstrates some standard real-time tests to evaluate the results. Once the emotional component is revealed you will see that the Setup language clearly points to a collection of specific events in which Budweiser meant good times. To be more specific in the session, any of those individual events could be addressed with Tell the Story Technique or the Movie Technique.

After addressing the emotional component, Tam uses some positive phrasing in the Setup to reframe his client's perspective. This approach is a more advanced EFT tool, and should generally be used only after the intensity has been released, just as Tam illustrates.

Budweiser and Emotions That Cause Addictions
by Tam Llewellyn

In EFT workshops, I often ask participants to bring addictive substances if they wish to see EFT remove the addiction. These usually involve sugar, chocolate, cigarettes, and coffee. However, at a recent workshop one of the participants came up with an unusual request.

Emma was not an alcoholic, in that she could do without alcohol and did for long periods, and she could take a social drink or two and not want more. Her problem was with Budweiser beer. Once she had a bottle she could not stop drinking it. She would drink and drink and drink until no more was available. To complicate matters, Emma wanted to lose her addiction to Budweiser beer but wanted to retain her liking for an occasional beer when it suited her.

I had never been asked to remove only part of an addiction. However, being willing to try anything once and with Gary Craig's words "Try it on everything!" ringing in my ears, I started the demonstration.

When a bottle of Budweiser was placed in front her, Emma immediately reported a 0-to-10 craving of 10. We tapped together for:

Even though I have a craving for this Budweiser beer, I deeply and completely accept and love myself.

We used the Reminder Phrase "Craving for Budweiser beer" while doing a full round of tapping. That first round reduced the craving to a 5, and after the second, it fell to a 2. I cracked the bottle open and the resulting hiss immediately took the craving back to 10. More rounds reduced it again to a 4 or 5, and even sipping the beer did not increase the craving, but it did not show any signs of falling, either.

It was Emma herself who made the breakthrough. She said, *"It's not the Budweiser beer, but the happy times I have associated with it."* That changed the line of the therapy and while I continued tapping around the points, she repeated my words:

Even though I loved those times, and want them back, and Budweiser beer reminds me of them, I deeply and completely accept and love myself as I am now.

Those times were great and so was the Budweiser beer, but I do not need it now. I can still remember and enjoy those times without the Budweiser beer.

I have a film running in my head called "Those Budweiser Beer Days" and I can remember them well. They were great.

Even though I think I need Budweiser beer to help me recover those times, I deeply and completely accept and love myself.

This work brought the craving level down to 2 and even sipping it did not bring it back up again. Emma said she could do without it and that anyway it tasted "strange," but she still had a little wish for it and those happy times.

This time we tapped while saying:

Even though I may need this Budweiser beer to recall those happy times, I choose to recall and enjoy them without Budweiser beer and I will be amazed and intrigued at how easy it is for me to rerun the film of those times (now re-titled simply "Happy Days") any time I wish. It is amazing that I do not need those days to come again — I am happy as I am now and I can still have lovely memories.

The craving level was down to zero and Emma was having uncontrolled fits of laughter.

Emma and the group were with us for a full week learning various therapies, and during that week I saw her drinking the occasional can of beer. But even when it was offered or even pressed on her, she never drank more than a sip of Budweiser, saying it was nowhere near as nice as other beers and really tasted a bit funny!

❖ ❖ ❖

Dr. Carol Solomon is up next to address an intense craving for ice cream. Once again, after peeling away a few surface layers, a very clear core issue emerges and presents an entire collection of specific events from child-hood. The connection between the events and the craving is so clear that you might wonder why Jannie didn't see it sooner. However, the human emotional framework can be tricky and elusive, so it's always good to have a tool like EFT and an experienced professional like Dr. Solomon to guide you through.

Detective Work for an Ice-Cream Addiction
by Dr. Carol Solomon

I teach a three-week teleclass on "EFT for Weight Loss," and I have people bring food to the first call so we can tap for cravings in the moment. After the first round of a recent class, almost everyone's craving was down, except one woman, "Jannie."

Jannie was tapping on her craving for ice cream, although she said she didn't bring it to the call because "unless someone delivered it as I dialed in, I would have eaten it the minute it came in the house!"

We tapped for cravings:

Even though I have this craving, I deeply and completely accept myself.

Even though I really want this food right now...

Even though I have this urge to eat...

We used the Reminder Phrase "this craving" on each tapping spot.

Her craving went from a 10 to a 2. But she was still worried that if someone put a bowl of ice cream in front of her, she would eat it, or that the craving could be triggered again in a stressful situation.

So we tapped more:

Even though I don't quite want to let it go, I deeply and completely accept myself.

Even though I'm afraid I'll still want it...

Even though I have these cravings that are triggered by stress...

Even though I want things I think I shouldn't have...

We changed Reminder Phrases as we tapped the EFT points down the body, saying: *these cravings...*

triggered by stress…I can't quite release it…I'm still hanging on…It's triggered by stress…I'm afraid I might still want it….I don't quite trust it yet…

Between the first and second call, Jannie did buy a quart of ice cream. It stayed in her refrigerator for 12 hours—11 hours and 59 minutes longer than usual! When she opened it, she just ate the cherries out and threw the rest away. She hasn't purchased any since and has no desire to get any.

On the third call, we tapped for specific events. Jannie came up with five events that had an emotional charge. These specific events all occurred when she was between seven and fifteen years old, and they all had to do with her parents and with her being denied something. For tapping during the class she picked "my mother eating ice cream every evening after dinner and I was not allowed any."

Jannie's mother was a 105-pound, 5-foot 2-inch, extremely beautiful woman who took very good care of herself and her home. She loved ice cream, so every evening she'd go to the freezer, pile ice cream into her salad bowl-sized dish, curl up at the end of the sofa, and eat it slowly bite by bite.

Jannie was not allowed to have any ice cream, ever, because she was chubby and "Jannie doesn't get sweets" was a house rule.

At some point in her life, Jannie made a decision, based on her interpretation of these childhood experiences, which she described in a letter to me following the class. She wrote:

Dear Carol,

When I decide to get ice cream, I always tell myself, "I deserve it"—not as a reward for anything, I just I deserve it. I never could figure this out because I am someone who is actually more humble than this and hugely grateful for my life and all I have been given.

Carol, this is phenomenal for me. It finally makes sense, perfect sense, actually. I did deserve it when those energies were stuck in the denial from my mother. When I tapped through all those issues around ice cream (being denied, feeling I deserved it, that I could have it anytime I wanted it, accepting my mother for who she was able to be and loving her anyway), I felt a great relief. I am at zero now with ice cream. And what I love most of all is that it finally makes sense to me! I remember that my mother always had gallons of ice cream around as well as all kinds of candy. I wondered why I didn't just go eat all that stuff anyway (I was not an obedient child). Then I remembered (funny, I had forgotten) that my parents had a lock on the freezer and a cupboard with a padlock in the kitchen to keep me out!

So I asked myself why have I never chowed down on all of those things all the time since I left home and have the freedom to do so? My eating is typically very healthy (I never keep anything in the house that is tempting to me) and although I am 20 pounds overweight, this is more due to orthopedic injuries and mid-life hormones than poor eating. In class #1, you said to me that I needed to trust myself. That resonated because, although I do really well, I strategically and stringently set up my environment to keep temptations out—always.

So my next revelation is about goodies locked up by my parents…I cannot be trusted, but I love all those goodies, so I essentially "lock up" all the goodies I'd love because I don't trust myself. So when you said I needed to trust myself, I actually felt your words in my heart right then, and now that I've figured it out, I feel such peace in knowing I can trust myself.

So Carol, this has been amazing for me and I thank you from the bottom of my heart. What I find with you is your insights and words bring normalcy to me and you make beautiful sense and connections and I feel all this so profoundly.

I thank you so much for pursuing this with me. I just read that victims will feel a sense of entitlement, and that resonates with me in thinking "I deserve this ice cream! Wow!"

In a four-month follow up, Jannie wrote to say that her results have held up, even under stressful circumstances. She tapped for a craving one more time, two weeks after the class ended. She wrote, "I must tell you that ice cream is so far out of the picture for me now. The true test has been my husband needing surgery and me needing "something" for comfort, but ice cream never even crossed my mind! I've been happily choosing berries, cherries, and grapes instead! This is an absolute miracle!!! Thank you, thank you!"

❀ ❀ ❀

Addictive cravings sometimes represent a crying out for love. You can often identify such cases when a few rounds of EFT directed at cravings have only minimal impact. That's because there's a bigger emotional need that drives them. In the next report, Gabriele Rother from Germany illustrates this concept beautifully.

Once again, global descriptions in the Setup peel away some layers so the core issue can come though. The extended Setup Phrases in the rest of the session are designed to increase the intensity of the anger by describing it in more detail. By focusing on the anger to this degree, the tapping can correct the related energy disruption more completely.

The Reminder Phrases are not distinguished from the Setup Phrases here, but you can assume that this language was used while tapping through the sequence and not just on the Karate Chop point.

Gabriele addresses several aspects along the way and then closes the session after resolving a specific event with her client's father.

A Chocolate Addiction
And the Reason Behind It

by Gabriele Rother

A woman called and asked me how she could tap for her intense craving for chocolate. She had experienced sudden attacks of cravings and was very angry at herself for eating the all of the chocolate in her possession at once.

We started tapping with the Setup Phrases:

Even though I have this ravenous appetite for chocolate, I deeply and completely accept myself.

Even though I don't like myself because I am so weak every time that I cannot resist...

Even though I am so angry afterwards...

Even though I have this addiction to chocolate...

This yearning for chocolate...

"What is your real yearning?" I asked. She replied, "Craving for security."

We tapped while saying:

Even though this yearning inside myself lets me take the chocolate...Chocolate means security for me. I never felt secure. I yearn for it so badly. I yearn for it forever. I know chocolate is not the same. Chocolate only reminds me of security and feeling safe.

After that round she felt very angry, and a lot of rage came up about the fact that she wasn't protected by her parents. They both were employed and didn't have time enough for her. This made her very upset. We tapped for:

This rage about my parents…I am still so furious, even though this happened a long time ago. I yearned so much for security and protection. I never got it. There was nobody protecting me. I had this yearning. This yearning is still there. The chocolate calms me down for a while but it comes back. And I am so angry about myself and about my parents. I am angry!

After this round she calmed down a bit, but it came to her that she was still angry with her aunt. She experienced abuse during a stay at her grandmother's and she told her aunt about that. But her aunt refused to listen to her and didn't take her seriously. That upset her. We tapped for:

Even though I feel this anger about my aunt… She didn't take me seriously. I am so angry about her. She didn't believe me. Nobody takes me seriously. That makes me so furious! I am mad with anger! But maybe my aunt was afraid of this man. I am still furious about her! Maybe she experienced something similar and had fears like me, but I am still furious…Nobody takes me seriously. But the chocolate takes me seriously. It is always there and gives me a good feeling. I wished I could have gotten that same feeling from my aunt.

After this round the anger about the aunt was gone. Now a sort of sadness and a feeling of anger came up about her father. He refused to take her home, and she was not able to tell him what happened with this man and that made her sad and angry at same time. We tapped:

My father…He didn't take me home. I am so angry about this. He does not love me. And I wasn't able to tell him what happened. Couldn't tell it to Grandma, neither to Dad, and my aunt refused to listen. I am so sad and so angry! But Dad wanted to protect me. He wanted to do his best for me. In his view, the best thing for me was to stay with my grandma. But he didn't know what happened there. He still loves me. And I couldn't tell him. If he knew what happened, he would have taken me home. But I couldn't tell him. At least it was OK. Nothing more happened. My aunt took care of me. At the end she protected me. I can let it go now and enjoy my chocolate without longing for it. I can enjoy the chocolate without being angry. I don't need to eat it up all at once. I can enjoy it that I feel safe now even without chocolate. I am protected and I am OK like I am.

Deep breath out. All of the anger and the sadness were gone. I asked her about her longing for chocolate. It was completely gone and she felt a deep release. This session took us about a quarter of an hour.

❀ ❀ ❀

Here's a brief idea from Dr. Deborah Miller that brings about big results for stubborn food cravings. Notice how her approach involves common-sense questions.

Finding Out What
Really Caused a Food Craving

by Dr. Deborah Miller

I enjoy how EFT allows one to get to the core reason for a food craving. This interesting story shows how well we hide the reasons.

I facilitate individual sessions and group classes titled "EFT Ideal Weight." It is a delightful way to look at the myriad causes of holding onto weight.

In one particular class dealing with food cravings, each person brought an item that she had cravings for. I asked each woman to look at the food item, smell it, and sense the emotions that came to the surface because I wanted them to identify what it was about the item that they craved. Was it the look, the taste, the texture?

With EFT the craving level dropped quickly for everyone except one woman. Her craving was for a specific type of bread. When I asked her what it was about the bread that she craved she admitted that it wasn't the bread. It was dunking the bread in milk. I asked her what it was about dunking the bread in milk that she enjoyed. She told me that it made the bread soft. The type of bread she craved is dry bread commonly used for dunking in milk or hot chocolate.

Then I asked her if there was something in her life that was hard that she wanted to make soft. Her eyes got wide and she stated that her husband was sometimes hard with her and she wished he'd be softer. From that moment on her craving level for the bread dropped to nothing. Since this session she hasn't had a craving for dunking bread in milk.

❊ ❊ ❊

German EFT'er Horst Benesch could not get a woman beyond her cookie craving until he persisted with questions and discovered a core issue. Once the core issue was collapsed with EFT, the cookie craving disappeared. This an important concept that all serious EFT'ers need to understand. Horst uses both the Karate Chop point and the Sore Spot while doing the Setup. You'll find the Sore Spot described in Appendix A.

The Core Issue Behind a Cookie Addiction

by Horst Benesch

In a recent EFT workshop I placed cookies in the middle of the tables and asked whether anyone irresistibly had to eat one of them. A 42-year-old woman said she could not imagine not eating this sugar-coated cookie. I let her smell and taste a bit, and she rated her craving at a 7.

We tapped for the craving, but there was no change. It remained a 7. We switched from the Karate Chop point to the Sore Spot with more emphasis, but no change. I let her bite a small piece again and asked her to describe what she sensed. She reported a certain pleasurable sense of melting in her mouth.

Even though I like this melting feeling in my mouth...

No change, still a 7.

I then asked her to describe this melting more exactly, asking what it felt like for her. She said, *"Smooth, warm, and sweet."* And she added: *"That is because my mother never nursed me."* I wanted to hook into this argument, but she refused and said it was just a joke. Nevertheless I asked her whether or not it was true. She conceded that her mother never had nursed her.

I told her to take this "joke" seriously, because maybe that is the way her unconscious tricked her. Thus we tapped on:

Even though my mother never did nurse me and even though I therefore miss this warm, smooth, and sweet sensation within my mouth...

After a whole round of the Basic Recipe, I let her taste it again. She was astonished and reported that this cookie tasted sweeter.

Another round of tapping, again tasting. Now she reported that it tasted unpleasantly sweet and she did not want to eat this cookie anymore. As a challenge I put cookies directly in front of her during the whole evening. She did not even feel a slight desire for them.

At the end of this group session I asked her again to have a little taste. She did not like it at all because it was too sweet.

❖ ❖ ❖

Carol Look has been a professional therapist for many years, and has an impressive record using EFT for addictions, weight loss, and the like. Over the years, she has identified several emotional "themes" that often contribute to addiction and weight loss, and in this case, we learn about grief.

In her article below, Carol tells us about how she addressed cravings at a workshop with a group of volunteers. Coincidentally, or maybe not, several of these volunteers had unresolved grief in their past. Once these stories are revealed by her volunteers, you can see how one traumatic event, left unresolved, can translate in to a lifetime of eating habits.

When applying EFT to several people at once, you often have to keep it global or general, and you may see that in Carol's Setup Phrases. This article can serve as a great illustration of how emotional issues connect to cravings, but as a follow-up on any of these issues, I would focus on the actual event of the loss with each volunteer.

Using the Client's Cravings

by Carol Look

Brenda attended my "EFT for Anxiety Relief" class at the National Guild of Hypnotists convention. As part of the agenda, I asked for volunteers for an in-class demonstration for food cravings and underlying feelings. Brenda was one of four volunteers.

She chose a bag of M&Ms from my pile of props and rated her craving for them as an 8 on the 0-to-10 point scale. Our first round of tapping was:

Even though I have these cravings, and I really love the way my favorite food tastes, I deeply and completely accept myself.

Each person's 0-to-10 craving rating decreased. One woman said her craving had gone down significantly and she was now thinking of the good times she had with her father. Brenda echoed this thought and reported feeling profound grief. She had lost her father when she was eight years old and her mother couldn't handle Brenda's grief and crying, so she gave Brenda food to shut her up.

All four volunteers associated their eating of junk foods with losses they had experienced.

Even though I feel deep grief, and I want to eat to cover it up, I deeply and completely accept myself.

Even though I feel these deep losses, and I want to stuff myself with food, I deeply and completely accept myself anyway.

Even though I feel abandoned because they left me, I deeply and completely accept my feelings.

The volunteers continued to unravel layers of sadness around the losses they had experienced. Brenda said that her craving for the M&Ms was going down dramatically, but her feelings of sadness were surfacing strongly. She told the class she had lost two children, a fiancé, and her favorite pet. She also reported having strong physical feelings of grief in her chest, which she described as "a bowling ball in my chest."

Even though I use the sweets to feel better, because I love how they make me feel, I choose to feel safe and comfortable without them.

Even though I can't get satisfied, I love myself anyway.

Even though sweets are the only things that make me feel better, I deeply and completely accept myself.

Brenda told the class that the "bowling ball feeling" in her chest, a heartache, was decreasing in intensity and moving down towards her solar plexus.

Even though I have suffered so many losses, I choose to feel accepting of myself and of them.

Even though I just want to be acknowledged for all my losses and how hard it's been, I deeply and completely love and accept my feelings.

Brenda said this one really "hit" her hard. She realized that all she had wanted was to be acknowledged for all the pain that she had been through. She told the class that everyone sees her as such a strong person and that they assume things come easily to her.

We tapped several more rounds on grief and being acknowledged.

We also tapped for Brenda's belief that whenever she gets close to someone, "they drop dead." Brenda said this last round released the tremendous pain she had been carrying around for so long. She heard herself say, *"You're right. I've suffered enough,"* and she felt free to let go of her deep grief at this point.

I talked to Brenda four weeks later to see how she was. She had been doing her own tapping during the first week but then stopped. She had not eaten any sweets since the class, including while she was on a week-long vacation in Florida. Ice cream used to be her favorite comfort food, and she hadn't had any in four weeks. On her birthday the week before she took one bite of birthday cake and didn't like it because it tasted too sweet! While in the class demonstration, Brenda used the bag of M&Ms as a symbol for all sweets in her life and was pleased that it had obviously worked for cake and ice cream as well.

Brenda said she had not gotten on the scale yet, but that several people told her she looked as if she had lost some weight.

She is ready now to deal fully with her weight issue and reported that the tapping came at exactly the right time in her life.

❅ ❅ ❅

There is a suggestion here that the results achieved in the workshop described above were more of a "good start" than a "miracle cure" and that Brenda should continue tapping. This is often the case when using global Setup Phrases instead of uncovering the specific events.

Here is another example of how an experience of grief or loss can eventually contribute to unhealthy eating habits. This next article by Melissa Derasmo is a must-read because it superbly illustrates how finding a core issue can collapse even the most stubborn challenges.

Her process provides a very good example of how everyday people without therapy experience can find their own underlying isues. Melissa immediately "got" that past events in her life were affecting her life in the present, so she committed herself completely without expecting any specific result right away. Once she was relieved of some baggage, she was able to tune into to the deeper issue comning forward.

Also notice the extent to which she tested her own results. Testing methods can dig up even more aspects and help you be much more thorough with EFT. As she discovers, it may be that one needs to tap on *what didn't happen* as well as what did.

EFT and My Sugar Addiction

by Melissa Derasmo

I was a confirmed sugar addict. Starting in my early twenties, I ate sugar at every opportunity. I would do anything I had to in order to get my "fix," including things I would rather not admit to, like stealing money if I didn't have any for chocolate or other sugar-rich things.

In a continuing effort to find the perfect diet, I somehow managed to discover EFT in August of 2007. I dove in and never looked back. I tapped for every single issue I could find, and I had a lot. I had inconsolable grief over my alcoholic mother dying when I was six, anger over being physically abused by a stepmother and sexually abused by *her* father, and then inconsolable grief over my father passing away when I was ten years old. These were big issues, but I was able to eliminate all their pain with EFT. I spent the next year working on my Personal Peace Procedure and tapping on everything I could come up with. But I still ate sugar uncontrollably.

Then on February 1, 2009, something happened that started me down the road to the answer. I was in Macy's shopping (which was my second favorite thing to do at that time) and suddenly out of nowhere a baby started screaming and crying. Well, my reaction to that was to get out of the room as fast as possible. My husband, who was with me at the time, turned to me and said, *"What is wrong with you?"* And it hit me. I thought *everyone* runs out of the room when there's a crying baby. I can't tolerate hearing babies cry. But no, apparently lots of people don't have this issue at all! And slowly the thought "bubbled up" for me—I can't tolerate the crying baby because *I* am the crying baby—the baby that wasn't taken care of—both while my mother was alive and after she died. So I went home and started to tap. This was a long session of working on every single thing I could come up with, and whether it was true or not did not matter. These thoughts were what I *believed* to be true.

Even though I'm so sad that my mother was too drunk to wake up and feed me...

too drunk to wake up and change my diapers...

too drunk to take care of me...

But more importantly, I realized that after she died she wasn't there to do all the things a daughter needs in life—and as I focused on what we had missed together, the tears came flooding out:

Even though I'm so sad my mother wasn't there to walk me to school,

tuck me in at night,

read me a story,

help me with my homework,

put my picture on the fridge,

congratulate me on my wonderful report card,

push me on the swing in the park,

listen to my heart aches,

play with me,

take me for my first bra,

make cookies with me,

tell me what a Tampax is,

help me plan my wedding,

tell me why I shouldn't marry that idiot,

hold her first granddaughter,

tell me what a great daughter I am,
…and lots, lots more.

What happened when it was all done was quite stunning. The first thing I noticed was total silence — the voice that would constantly scream out for sugar was completely silent. So I started to test. At work I walked by my co-worker's office and the ton of chocolate on her desk — *nothing*. I went by the vending machines — *nothing*. I went to the supermarket and walked down candy aisle — *nothing*. I picked up some chocolate, smelled it, had zero desire for it, put it down, and walked away. If you are a sugar addict, you will understand that that was nothing less than a miracle. The next morning I thought perhaps I had been abducted by aliens and exchanged for an addiction-free person — someone who is "normal." I was quite unsettled about it but willing to accept that whatever happened, it was good. And while it hasn't been a terribly long time, I remain completely addiction-free weeks later. The endless, relentless "pull" that would force me to eat is completely gone. Today I eat "normally" — I make low-calorie balanced meals and I'm perfectly OK with them. I'm happy with one serving. I can watch others eat cake, cookies, and candy without any issue at all. It doesn't bother me. I simply don't want what they have.

Looking back, I can see the clue my subconscious was trying to give me with the crying baby who was always there. I didn't understand what it meant so I just ignored it. And as I now lose weight effortlessly,

I hope that others will find this information useful. It may be that one needs to tap on *what didn't happen* as well as what did.

Since first collapsing the "baby crying" issue, I have now been three months without any sugar cravings and I have lost 38 pounds.

❊ ❊ ❊

Melissa discovered both physical and sexual abuse in her past, which are very traumatic experiences that often lead to overeating. However, don't assume that only abuse survivors can relate to her process. Believe it or not, many people have been just as traumatized by a playground humiliation or by being dumped by a first love. If it was really painful for you, it can still be affecting you, so tap on whatever memories show up.

4

Are You Getting the
Results You Want?

By now you have probably tried the EFT Basic Recipe, or maybe some creative variations, on a few of your strongest cravings. With any luck, you have also uncovered some important specific events or possibly some limiting beliefs. No matter what you have tried, this is a good time to evaluate your progress and decide where to go next.

If you have not yet tried EFT, I suggest you try it now because the next session will provide some direction based on your results—or lack thereof. Do a few basic rounds on your strongest craving, then follow the guidelines below.

Results and Refinements

There are five possible outcomes after doing a full round of EFT.

1. The craving or discomfort level improves or goes away completely.

2. The location of a physical symptom, such as a headache or other pain, moves to another part of the body, even if it only moves an inch or two.

3. The quality of the craving or discomfort changes.

4. The craving or discomfort level increases.

5. Nothing happens.

I'll cover what to do about each of these possibilities in detail, but please note that:

All of the changes in items 1 through 4 are evidence that EFT is working for you.

1. What should you do if the craving or discomfort level improves or goes away completely? If the craving or discomfort goes away completely, you are done. You're one of our well-known "one-minute wonders," and while you may find it surprising, this is a frequent occurrence. Enjoy the results and get on with your life.

If the craving or discomfort improves but doesn't go to zero, do more EFT rounds until it reaches zero or plateaus at some improved level. If it plateaus and three or four more EFT rounds don't result in relief, you can assume that "nothing more will happen" and go to item 5 below.

If the craving or discomfort disappears but resurfaces at another time, this is evidence that more EFT is necessary. It would be a mistake to conclude that EFT "didn't work" because it obviously did. Our bodies give us many valuable messages (if we are listening) and sometimes a single symptom can have several causes. You can try more rounds of standard EFT and, eventually, the discomfort or craving may subside permanently. If not, just assume that "nothing more will happen" and go to item 5 below.

2. What should you do if the location of a physical symptom moves to another part of the body, even if it only moves an inch or two? Sometimes while tapping for a specific food craving, a person will suddenly feel nauseated or develop a headache or feel pain or discomfort somewhere in the body. (See an example on pages 95–96). Any new symptom or movement of a symptom is cause for optimism because it suggests that the original problem has been alleviated in favor of a new discomfort that now gets your attention. It could also mean that the original discomfort had an emotional cause that was "alleviated in the background" and the new discomfort or craving is evidence of a new emotional cause. In either case, start over with EFT at the new location just as though it is a brand new condition—because it is.

If the symptom moves again, then keep "chasing" it until the discomfort level falls to zero. If you get stuck on a symptom that doesn't move or if you don't get relief after three or four diligent rounds of EFT, then assume that "nothing more will happen" and proceed to item 5 below.

3. What should you do if the quality of the symptom changes from, let's say, a sharp pain to a dull ache, or from a throb to a tingle…and so on? This is similar to item 2 above except the symptom changes nature or quality instead of location. Any such quality change is cause for optimism because it suggests that the original condition has been altered.

In this case, start over with EFT as though this altered version is a new condition. Keep doing EFT rounds on any future altered symptoms until the discomfort level falls to zero. If you get stuck on an altered symptom that doesn't move or if you don't get relief on it after three or four diligent rounds of EFT, then assume that "nothing more will happen" and proceed to item 5 below.

4. What should you do if the discomfort level or craving increases? Although it doesn't happen often, I have certainly seen cases where such levels increased after one or two rounds of EFT. Many healing responses triggered by other therapies show signs of getting worse (they call it a "healing crisis") before getting better.

Three or four more rounds of EFT will usually "turn the corner" and launch noticeable relief. If not, or if the relief plateaus at a level above zero, then assume that "nothing more will happen" and proceed to item 5.

5. What should you do if nothing happens? The high likelihood here is that unresolved emotional issues are major contributors to the craving or discomfort you feel.

So now we need to search for emotional factors and apply EFT to them. Since we have so many differing emotional histories, this bit of detective work has to be customized to you. I usually do this by asking questions. Here's one:

> *If there was a specific emotional event contributing to this craving or this feeling of discomfort, what could it be?*

The beautiful thing about this question is that it often points to a vital emotional cause even if it doesn't seem that way at first. Your system has a way of knowing what is going on even if you see no realistic link. For example, your craving for vanilla pudding may seem to have no connection to the memory of your third grade teacher ridiculing you in front of the class. That's OK, just use EFT on that memory with a Setup Phrase like:

Even though Mrs. Johnson humiliated me in third grade...

Do this for as many rounds as it takes to bring your current emotional intensity on this event down to zero. When finished, you are likely to notice complete relief from the craving. If not, ask the question again and use EFT on the resulting emotional issue. Repeated efforts at this are likely to have two benefits: the emotional events will lose their sting (probably permanently) and your craving or discomfort should fade considerably.

Another good question is:

If you could live your life over again, what person or event would you just as soon skip?

This question is more general than the previous one but its answer usually leads to important specific events that need collapsing. For example, if your answer to the above is "My brother Jake," then you can break down your experience with Jake into all the specific events you have had with him that left you feeling angry, frustrated, afraid, etc.

With these two questions, you can uncover and resolve important issues that limit your life and cause you pain and/or other symptoms. That's very useful.

One point, though. You MUST come up with an answer to these questions or they will be useless. A response like "I don't know" is unacceptable. If you really don't know, use the first guess that comes to mind. If you don't even have a guess, then *MAKE ONE UP!*

Often a made-up issue is as good as or better than a real one. That's because it still came from you and thus it isn't totally fictitious. It still has your experiences and emotions embedded within it and it can even blend several "forgotten issues" together in a useful way.

When EFT Doesn't Work

When progress with EFT seems stopped—or it seems as though "it doesn't work"—EFT is usually not the problem. Rather, the reason for the lack of progress can most often be traced to the user's inexperience.

Why do I say this? Because those who master EFT don't miss very often.

They not only get their share of "one minute wonders" but impressive progress is also made for just about any problem with an emotional cause, including many physical ailments.

In those cases where the masters are stumped, however, they don't point the finger at EFT for "not working." Rather, the masters ask themselves questions like:

"What's in the way here?"

"What have I not seen yet?"

"What core issue have I been unable to find?"

After asking myself those questions, session after session, for many years now, here is a list of the most common reasons why EFT hasn't produced the expected results.

- The problem is being approached too globally.

- The Setup was not performed completely enough.

- You have switched aspects (and may be unaware of the improvement on the previous aspect).

- You may need help from a friend or professional with a different perspective.

- You may need the full Basic Recipe including the 9 Gamut Procedure and EFT's finger points (see Appendix A).

- You may need more instruction, so consider EFT trainings, books and DVDs.

By far, the most common reason, especially with beginners, is that the problem is being approached too globally. Next, I have included an article from the EFT website with further insight on being as specific as possible and finding those individual events.

The Importance of Being Specific

This tutorial should be read several times. It is that important.

Why? Because it addresses one of the most common errors made by newcomers to EFT. Once this is corrected, your results will have much greater consistency and many of your "difficult cases" will melt away quite easily.

The problem is that most clients tend to see their issues through "global glasses." That is, they describe their issues using broad labels which, to them, seem very specific. Examples might be:

> *"I just don't feel very good about myself."*
>
> *"My father always abused me."*
>
> *"My mother never gave me the love I should have had."*
>
> *"I don't do very well with relationships."*
>
> *"I'm easily rejected."*

Each of these, and countless more like them, are like emotional forests made up of specific trees (negative events) which contribute to the overall problem. Using EFT on the globally stated problem is like trying to chop down an entire forest with one swing of the axe. If you address the problem in this way, you will probably make some progress each time you swing. However, compared to the enormity of the forest, the progress is not likely to be noticed and thus the client will probably claim "no result," or you might erroneously consider the person to be hopelessly Psychologically Reversed, or you might erroneously conclude that the person is beset with energy toxins, or you might give up and think EFT "doesn't work" or…or…or.

Instead of using EFT on an issue like, *"Even though I'm easily rejected...,"* it is best to break down the globally stated problem into specific events such as:

Even though my third-grade teacher embarrassed me in front of the class...

Even though I felt so left out when my father didn't attend my high school graduation...

Even though my high school sweetheart said, "I've grown tired of you..."

Even though I was sent to my room for the whole day on Thanksgiving at age eight...

Even though Mom told me, "You'll never get married unless you are thin like your sister..."

These are the **true contributors** to the *"I'm easily rejected"* issue. They represent the **foundation** of the problem. The feeling of rejection is but a symptom of these underlying specific causes. Stated differently, if we didn't have these specific causes, how could we possibly feel rejection? The answer is that we couldn't because there would be no prior experience by which to measure a current "rejection."

So...we need to neutralize these causes by using EFT on individual trees. When we do, several benefits occur.

1. You can easily recognize whenever EFT has eliminated a negative tree from your forest. You may start with an intensity of 7–10 for a given event and end with an intensity of zero. This is clearly noticeable and thus substantially improves your confidence in the method.

2. Each tree that is removed thins out the forest. This allows you to walk through the forest with more ease instead of constantly bumping into "rejection trees." The sting of rejection becomes less and less.

3. An important generalization effect occurs. The various "rejection trees" tend to have some common themes among them so that removing one tree has an effect on the remaining ones. Often, we can remove five or ten trees and then watch the whole forest fall.

I cannot overemphasize the importance of being specific. It often spells the difference between dramatic success and apparent failure.

Weight Loss and Tail-enders

Another way to uncover important issues, limiting beliefs, and specific events related to your weight is to use an affirmation process that will trigger "tail-enders." Tail-enders are the "yes, but" statements that contradict and sabotage your new goals.

For example, if you ask your system to confirm something that isn't currently true, such as, "I now look like a swimsuit model," your mind will instantly begin screaming its objections. Here's how to take advantage of these objections and make them work for you.

My normal weight currently fluctuates around 165 pounds. That's what I've weighed for a long time, but at one point in my life I gained a lot of weight. That wasn't surprising considering that almost every day I ate a large package of Oreo cookies and half a gallon of ice cream at one sitting. Eventually I got up to 195 pounds.

This was in the early 1980s and EFT didn't yet exist. To lose the extra weight, I set a goal for myself and repeated a short, simple weight-loss affirmation many times a day. That affirmation went like this: "My normal weight is 160 pounds, and that's what I weigh." Although it took me six months of ups and downs, gains and losses, and an unusual amount of determination, my weight eventually dropped back down to 160 pounds and stayed there. Affirmations were the best tool I knew back then, and they have been known to produce respectable results, but if EFT had been available, I could have saved myself a lot of time and effort. Now you can, too.

These days, I use affirmations as a way to identify the core issues behind challenges like weight loss. If you're like most of us, saying a simple affirmation will bring up a trail of negative self-talk that ensures you will never reach your goal.

For example, if your goal weight is 125 pounds, you might use the following statement:

> *My normal weight is 125 pounds and that's what I weigh.*

Try this now by filling the blank with your ideal weight and saying it out loud with as much conviction as you can muster:

> *My normal weight is _____ pounds and that's what I weigh.*

Now listen to what happens on the inside. When you declare a reality that is not currently true, your conflicting issues will often present some opposition, also known as negative self-talk or tail-enders. You might hear something like:

> *No way…look at the scale.*
>
> *It isn't safe to be that thin.*
>
> *I'm afraid of being hungry.*
>
> *My friends or family won't like me.*
>
> *I won't be able to complain anymore.*
>
> *I can't afford new clothes.*
>
> *I don't trust skinny people.*
>
> *I'll never lose weight.*
>
> *I'll always be fat.*
>
> *I can never be skinny.*
>
> *Look at this cellulite!*
>
> *Losing weight is just too difficult.*

Unaddressed, tail-enders have the power to sabotage any goal you try to achieve. On the bright side, tail-enders also point directly to issues you can disarm with EFT, thus removing their power from your weight loss process.

For example, if the tail-ender you heard was "My friends won't like me," you can bet there have been events in your life that helped you come to that conclusion. Take some time to review your experiences and tap on any events that might be related. Maybe your mother made fun of the skinny kid who lived next door or you heard your friends judge thin people on TV. Anything like this could contribute to your resistance to losing weight, but using EFT for those events can release their intensity and provide the freedom you need to reach your goal.

Once you identify a specific event that may be contributing to your issue with weight, simply tap the points while telling the story of that event until its emotional intensity disappears. To be more effective, identify which emotions you experienced during the event and address them individually:

> *Even though I felt humiliated when my mother said that, I deeply and completely accept myself.*

Use *"this humiliation"* as your Reminder Phrase.

Once the emotional intensity for *humiliation* is released, substitute anger, hopelessness, or any other feeling you experienced and address it next.

There are several common "themes" for people who can't lose weight. For some, weight is a shield that protects them from having to do certain things, like socializing or being intimate. Others have a painful association with exercise or feeling hungry. Most often, for myself included, food can be a form of self-medication, something we indulge in the way other people indulge in cigarettes, alcohol, or other addictions. We do it because it makes us feel better—at least temporarily—by relieving or suppressing at least some of our stress, anxiety, fear, anger, or other damaging emotions. If any of these themes resonate with you, use them to identify the individual events that are still affecting you and address them with EFT.

Another way to find core issues is to ask yourself the simple question:

If there were an emotional reason why I can't lose weight, what would it be?

You can also complete the following sentences:

If I reach my goal weight of 130 pounds, the consequences would be _____.

In order to lose that much weight I would have to _____.

Losing weight would be nice, but what I really want is _____.

Losing weight reminds me of _____.

These queries can bring up a whole daisy chain of events, beliefs, attitudes, and other tail-enders that are restricting your life and showing up on your body as excess pounds. Whether you use challenging questions, affirmations, or some other process to find these issues, break them down into specific events and tap them away with EFT. You'll notice a greater sense of overall relief with each event you address and soon your excess need for food will start to fade.

More Helpful Hints

If your issue is stubborn and just won't budge, or if you are ready for even better results, here are some more approaches you can try.

- **Tap with a friend:** Whether it's the feeling of support, an objective outside perspective, or the increased motivation, tapping with a friend can often make a big difference in your results. Find a friend who also wants to lose weight and then schedule an hour together once or twice a week. Work together to find the underlying events, then take turns using the Tell the Story Technique to address them.

- **Break out the oldies and the photo albums:** What are your favorite songs from the "good old days"? Do you remember any that still make you cry? What about the yearbooks and old family photos? Chances are, your old collections of music and photographs will remind you of important emotional events that you might overlook otherwise.

- **Adding emphasis:** When your normal tapping rounds haven't shown any progress, try raising your voice to add some emphasis. Shout the Setup Phrase, especially the "I deeply and completely accept myself" part. Say it with as much emotion as possible and see if that makes a difference.

- **What words are you using?** If you feel intimidated because you're unsure of what words to use, then it's likely that you are not being specific enough. Ask yourself a few more questions and do a little more detective work. Once you find something specific, like an event from the past, then use the Tell the Story Technique and just describe it as though you were telling it to a friend. Otherwise, go back to the default "Even though I have this _____, I deeply and completely accept myself."

- **Testing, testing, testing:** Whether you're working on a craving or a more general belief about food, putting yourself in the actual situation is a very powerful way to dig up contributing factors. What are the times of day, emotional events, or particular foods that make you feel the most like eating? In those moments, try *not eating* and take a few moments to see what emotions or memories are there waiting for you. Going to your parents' house for dinner might also bring up childhood food memories that need attention.

- **Daily tapping:** If all of this detective work and bothersome memories are more than you want to deal with right now, just try tapping every day. You can tap on whatever emotional events happen during the day, or just do a few rounds on "Even though I have this weight loss issue…" It is a global, longer-term approach, but if you tap your meridian points several times a day for a month, you may be surprised by the results.

- **Personal Peace Procedure:** I always recommend the Personal Peace Procedure as a fantastic way to start making significant shifts in your life. Rather than doing all the detective work, you can sit down once and make a list of past events that were less than pleasant. Then simply resolve one or more each day with EFT. The complete instructions were provided in Chapter One (see page 57).

- **Easy EFT:** This is a tap-along procedure that you can use with EFT videos. Just identify a problem that you want to work on, pop a DVD in the player, and tap along with the session. You can do this once a day or as often as you like. The sessions are entertaining and you get to "borrow benefits" for yourself. Please review the complete instructions in Appendix B before getting started.

- **Hire a practitioner:** The EFT website provides a list of experienced EFT professionals who resolve these issues for a living. Many of them list weight loss as a specialty, but you will get good results from anyone who can uncover your core issues. Keep in mind that EFT is just as effective over the phone, so I would suggest working with one who seems best suited for you, rather than the one located closest to you.

The following case from Michelle Hardwick shows how easily tapping can be worked into your daily routine.

Sugar Cravings Subside with Persistent EFT
by Michelle Hardwick

I encourage all my clients to use EFT on a regular basis. This allows them to feel empowered and to be in charge of their own growth, change, and healing and to have the tools to continue to make changes throughout the rest of their lives. I encourage everyone to tap. I tell them that I tap in the car, when on the toilet, in the shower, waiting for planes/trains/buses etc., in fact *anywhere!* I give plenty of examples so that clients can see how EFT can be a part of their everyday lives, not just once a week or fortnight when they see an EFT practitioner!

Recently, I encouraged one of my clients, who was suffering from extreme sugar cravings that were completely out of control, to tap on a regular basis, whenever she thought of sugar, whenever she thought of overeating, whenever the urge or craving hit, during it, after it if she forgot to tap, and whenever she felt fearful or worried about a craving happening again in the future. I asked her to think about as many other aspects about the craving that she could think of and tap on them. I explained that the more specific she could be in that moment about the craving, the better.

She returned for a follow-up session this week, saying, "Wow! It really works! I tapped during the ad breaks while watching TV. I just put the TV on mute and did a good couple of rounds of tapping and when my program came back on, I turned the sound back on and continued watching. There's not a night I didn't do that tapping."

And what happened to her sugar craving? She went 13 days without feeling it at all! That same craving had been out of control for the past five weeks. We still have a little way to go, but we made major progress after just one session! She was thrilled with the change.

So for those of you who say there's not enough time in your day to tap, I suggest that you first tap on the belief of having "no time to tap," and how about doing it during your ad breaks? Happy tapping!!

❖ ❖ ❖

5

Exploring
Underlying Issues

Every once in a while, someone tries the basic EFT formula and gets immediate, lasting results. The problem disappears in a single session and never comes back. One-minute wonders can and do happen, even with over-whelming cravings and an inability to lose weight. But in many cases, at some point after basic EFT reduces or eliminates a symptom or problem, it comes back. If this happens to you, don't assume that EFT didn't work. EFT worked fine for the problem you treated, but now a new aspect has presented itself, which just means there's more to do.

In this next example, Tam Llewellyn of the U.K. helps a woman lose weight when he discovers an aspect that she wasn't aware of.

Finding the Root of the Problem

by Tam Llewellyn

When we use EFT it is essential that we tap on the correct problem. This may seem obvious, but it is very easy to miss the major aspect of the problem — the one which is really driving the discomfort.

Finding the "correct" Setup Phrase is essential. I feel that when EFT fails to solve the issue, by far the most likely reason is that we have chosen the wrong aspect of the problem, or even the wrong problem altogether. Often the problem seems obvious, but in these cases we should be especially on our guard. If it is so obvious, why was it not identified and treated long ago?

In a case that illustrates this point, a middle-aged woman had a number of physical and emotional problems that all appeared to relate to her being grossly overweight. The cause of her excess weight was obvious — she ate too much and exercised too little.

We worked on various aspects of her over-eating and found that they were all related to incidents in her past. These were soon dealt with using EFT and her weight dropped a little. However, she eventually admitted to being "hooked" on Crunchie Bars (a chocolate bar available in U.K.). Her craving for them was removed using EFT to the extent that the smell and very idea of them revolted her. The job appeared to be done and I left a month's gap until her next appointment, expecting her to lose a considerable amount of weight by then and to be ready to work with me on other problems.

But a month later she returned, still overweight and still eating Crunchie Bars. She hated the smell and taste of the Crunchie Bars but was still eating four or five a day! We spent a long session exploring this aspect and I eventually discovered that many years ago the client had been in a "Weight Watchers' Club" using a strict diet plan. Crunchie Bars were included in the diet as a reward if one complied with the diet. They had been associated in the client's mind as a reward and she still felt happy and rewarded eating them — even though they tasted awful!

We could have tapped forever on her excessive weight and the problems it was causing, but we would likely have gotten little result. As soon as the link between Crunchie Bars and the feeling of reward was tapped away, her weight and related problems disappeared.

❄ ❄ ❄

While this next article by Emily P. of Canada doesn't go into specific EFT tapping details, it does an excellent job of getting behind the type of issues that cause people to carry extra weight. It also describes how EFT success stories can inspire students and practitioners alike in their use of EFT for problem solving.

Persistent EFT for Chubby Issues

by Emily P.

I have always had a serious propensity for all foods sweet and creamy—and a reputation for having an unquenchable appetite for such things. Even when I was able to temporarily eliminate my sugar addiction through EFT last year, I always seemed to sabotage myself by indulging in ice cream or chocolate. So, when I read an article in the EFT newsletter about the core issue behind a woman's cookie craving (the fact that her mother had never nursed her), a big light bulb went off! My mother had tried to nurse me but wasn't able to. Unfortunately, she didn't realize this until I lost a lot of weight and became rather emaciated. I was horribly unhappy and colicky, and it wasn't until I was put on formula that I became a happier and (very) chubby baby.

As long as I can remember, I have struggled with my weight and my love of sweets. I decided to try EFT on my similar issue, linking it to the idea that I associate sweet and creamy foods with the comfort and security I never got as a baby because I was starving and denied the food I so desperately needed. However, that didn't seem to work. In fact, over the course of the two days after I applied EFT, I actually craved sweet flavors and creaminess even more than I had in the recent past! I couldn't figure out what was going on, but I went back to the *EFT Manual* and started to read about Psychological Reversal. It made sense as the reason for my stalled progress, but what could I do about it?

I suddenly realised that the sweet and creamy cravings were also connected to my ongoing body weight issue—I work out intensively at the gym five or six days a week and have significantly increased my muscle mass, but my metabolism has remained stubbornly sluggish, and I have lost very little fat regardless of my workouts. I became conscious that many people in my life—family, teachers, friends—had always called me smart, not athletic.

The message I received was that I could never be lean, strong, and beautiful. I started to tap on that, and feelings rose to the surface, one after the other. First, I started laughing about the silly people telling me these things. Then I started to feel really angry! What right did they have to pigeonhole me into not being the "athletic type"? To always remember me as being chubby (and comment on it when they saw me after a few years away), even when they'd seen me thin at other times in my life? Vivid memories about my mother telling me how beautiful I could have looked in my prom dress—"if you could just lose five more pounds, it would be perfect." I started shouting as I tapped, and my eyes started to tear, thinking about all the hurt that those statements had done to me over the years. And then suddenly that started to fade, and I started to embrace the idea that I could be lean, strong, and beautiful.

I could erase those harmful words and forgive all the people who had contributed them. I started to smile and feel strong and confident in myself, and the best part was the overall sense of relief I was starting to feel. While I had already embraced that I am very strong, I could finally imagine my body being lean, and I could imagine feeling beautiful because of it, which is an image I had never been able to tangibly visualize before.

By the time I finished, I was feeling lighter, I was smiling, and I was barely able to picture a piece of chocolate in my mind!

* * *

The Comfort Zone

The *comfort zone* is a critical concept within all performance pursuits. This is the mental place where one subconsciously believes he or she "belongs." It is what keeps a situation at its current level and, without properly addressing it, any improvements one might achieve are not likely to be lasting.

Like a thermostat that keeps a room within a comfortable temperature range, our condition fluctuates within certain comfort zones. Ironically, most comfort zones aren't really comfortable, especially when we want to make changes. It's more accurate to call them *familiar* zones.

To properly enhance one's performance, condition, or situation, two factors should be addressed.

1. You must move the comfort zone to better levels, and
2. You must address the specific impediments to performance that need improvement.

Here are some examples of Setup Phrases that can help people involved in many different activities move beyond their present comfort zones. Please note that they all include a statement about the new or desired level of performance, whether it's an improved golf score, better grades, or the person's income. This is important in order to move mentally into a new vision of themselves.

Even though I'm not comfortable at the thought of golfing in the high 70s and may think I don't belong there, I deeply and completely accept myself.

Even though I think I am capable of being an A student in math but have never been above a B yet...

Even though the violin doesn't dance in my hands like it does in my dreams...

Even though I have yet to earn $200,000 per year...

Even though, as a speaker, I feel uptight and have yet to have fun with my audience...

Even though I just don't feel attractive and don't have the same outgoing charisma as [pick a role model]...

Even though I go "gulp" instead of flowing freely when I try to sing that high note in [name a song]...

Even though writer's block seems to be always with me instead of ideas flowing out of me like a fountain...

These go on endlessly and, of course, you must customize your approach to fit the situation. The idea is to move to a new mental image of yourself in which you see yourself as "belonging" at this new level.

Truly skilled EFT artists do a thorough job with their clients' comfort zones. They dig for the *specific events* underlying their clients' less-than-optimum performance levels and use EFT to obliterate these barriers.

When it comes to weight loss, your comfort zone is the weight range you usually maintain. It is easy for most people to lose a little weight, but when the weight loss goal is substantial, it's often outside the person's comfort zone. When that happens, self-sabotage enters the picture and the subconscious mind conspires with energy blocks, tail-enders, and negative self-talk to prevent the desired weight loss.

One way to use EFT to expand your weight-loss comfort zone is to choose a goal weight that is (as far as your mind is concerned) within the realm of possibility. Just as a golfer whose usual score is over 100 will find it hard to imagine shooting in the low 60s, someone who is 100 pounds overweight will find it hard to imagine easily reaching his or her goal weight.

But if the golfer sets a more modest goal, like shooting in the low 90s or high 80s, and if the overweight person decides to lose 20 or 30 pounds rather than 100 pounds, the subconscious mind is more likely to cooperate and less likely to generate self-sabotage. Many weight-loss success stories began with modest goals that, once achieved, led to revised and more ambitious goals.

EFT Setups that can help expand your weight-loss comfort zone include:

> *Even though I can't imagine ever being a size 12 again, I deeply and completely accept myself.*

Even though it's been a long time since I weighed 150 pounds, I would like to love and forgive my body and my past food choices.

Even though I have yet to lose five pounds, let alone 25 or 50, I deeply and completely accept myself anyway.

Even though it will be easier for me to climb stairs and get the exercise I need if I lose weight, I can move forward in a new direction starting now.

Even though I haven't been in a swimsuit for years, and the thought of wearing one in public is a real stretch, I would love to start swimming again.

Even though I'm not used to thinking of weight-loss as effortless or enjoyable, I know that with EFT, just about anything is possible.

Whenever you incorporate a goal into your EFT Setup Phrases, be on the alert for tail-enders, the "yes, but" statements that interfere with your progress. As soon as they come to mind, follow them back to specific events and the core issues they created. Becoming an EFT detective will help you quickly and efficiently clear away the mental and energy blocks that can otherwise undermine your best-laid plans.

Detective Skills

Core issues behind weight gain and cravings are often clever about hiding, so being a good detective is an EFT asset. Finding them can be as simple as asking yourself a few good questions:

What does this craving remind me of?

When was the first time I felt this way? And what was happening in my life at that time?

If there is a deeper emotion underlying this situation, what might it be?

Who or what is behind my weight gain?

If I could live my life over again, what person or event would I prefer to skip?

If there were a consequence for losing weight, what would it be?

If there were a benefit to keeping the weight, what would it be?

How do I feel just before I get the munchies? Exhausted, stressed, frustrated, sad, empty, angry, insecure, alone, disappointed...? And what does that feeling remind me of?

Once you have an answer to any of these questions, continue asking *"Why?"* or *"What's behind that?"* until you find unresolved specific events.

If you can't think of anything, you can try a few rounds of EFT on something global to remove a few emotional layers and see if anything new pops up.

Even though I have this weight issue and I don't know what is causing it, I deeply and completely accept myself.

For Reminder Phrases try *"This weight issue"* or *"Whatever is causing my weight issue."*

Even though food makes me feel better and I don't understand why, I deeply and completely accept myself.

For Reminder Phrases try *"Food makes me feel better"* and/or *"I wonder why."*

Even though I eat when I'm not hungry, and I know there is an emotional cause, I deeply and completely accept myself.

For Reminder Phrases try *"This emotional cause"* or *"I'm not even hungry."*

If you're still not able to come up with an event, memory, or connection, no problem. Just make something up. As I often say, a made-up example can work even better than an actual event or memory.

Tell yourself, *"If I had to imagine an event that could contribute to my weight problem, it would go something like this..."* Then use whatever event you create.

As soon as you have something, real or imaginary, that's connected in any way to your cravings or weight gain, create a short or long Setup Phrase around it and begin tapping.

These specific events are the building blocks underneath the bigger global issues. By dealing with them one at a time, they are easier to manage, and you can monitor your progress along the way. In addition, by going all the way to the foundation of the issue, you can start releasing these building blocks one by one until the global issue collapses.

Two points about this idea deserve special attention:

1. There can be hundreds or thousands of such specific events underlying a larger issue and thus, theoretically, addressing all of them can be a tedious process. Fortunately, you do not have to address every specific event to collapse the larger issue. You can usually do the job by collapsing somewhere between five and twenty of its table legs. This is because there is usually a commonality or "general theme" among those specific events. After EFT appropriately collapses a few of the table legs, a generalization effect occurs that serves to collapse the rest.

2. Remember that each specific event is likely to have an assortment of aspects, so address them separately and measure your progress on them one by one. Aspects can be the different emotions you felt during an event, the various emotional crescendos, or anything else that you would consider to be a "part" of your reaction to the event. An example given in Chapter One *(the time my mother left me in the shopping mall when I was in second grade)* is a good illustration. Why? Because the event probably contains many aspects such as *the fear of being all by myself; the fear of all those big adults walking around me; the "I-don't-care look" in mother's eyes when I arrived home; the guilt I felt for what I might have done to cause this;* and so on. Each of those pieces is an aspect all by itself and should be addressed separately.

To be as thorough as possible with any specific event, use the Tell the Story Technique until you can tell the complete story without any emotional spikes.

❊ ❊ ❊

In this insightful report by John Garrett, a woman taps through her tangled emotions toward her sister, thus freeing herself to lose weight. For your own practice, look for the Setup Phrases and identify which ones could be pursued as specific events and which ones represent global emotions.

Emotional Issues Had to Go First

by John R. Garrett

A client, I'll call her Tina, came to me frustrated by the lack of progress with her weight issue. She was morbidly obese and had been dieting and working out intensely for six weeks with nothing much to show for her efforts.

The day before she came to me, she experienced a confrontation with her older sister, Liz, who was a competitive body builder and personal trainer. She had asked Liz about what to do for sore knees from doing leg presses and got a lengthy lecture about her past eating habits. Liz chastised her for food choices as far back as when they were young children and criticized her for allowing her son to also become overweight. She prefaced these statements with, "I don't mean to hurt your feelings, but..."

My client was very hurt by Liz's unsolicited criticism and became defensive and angry at Liz's response. Liz also responded with anger and defensiveness, which created a huge, ugly confrontation.

By the time Tina expressed her feelings, she was ready to give up on the idea of ever being thin and fit, and she felt she just had to accept her sister's judgment. The fact that she could not remember what she had for breakfast while Liz claimed to remember what she had eaten as a child 35 years earlier made her incredibly self-conscious. She felt shame at being told to stop blaming genetics for her weight issues (they came from a long line of large people) and was hurt at being told that she and her son were fat simply because they ate too much.

My client was angry, but even more, she felt embarrassed and defeated. She carried intense guilt about her teenage son's weight issues and was horrified that he seemed to be following in her overweight footsteps. The confrontation with her sister confirmed her guilt, and it robbed her of energy and momentum to continue working out and following a diet program. In tears, she was ready to give up.

She decided to work with me not to resolve weight issues but to deal with the visions she had after the confrontation. She was so disturbed by these visions that she knew instinctively there was more going on than simple overeating.

Tina had thrown herself into her bed in tears after the confrontation with her sister. She dozed but didn't sleep. While in what she described as an Alpha or self-hypnotic state, she envisioned herself as an infant, with Liz, who was three years older, standing by her crib. Liz reached through the bars on the crib and pinched Tina hard on her arms and legs, intentionally making Tina cry. Her sense was that Liz was intensely jealous of the new baby and wanted to hurt her for disrupting her life and her relationship with their mother. Tina then had repeated visions of her sister covering her mouth and nose with her hand, trying to suffocate her. Several visions surfaced of Liz placing a pillow over Tina's face, which caused Tina to struggle with panic.

These visions startled and terrified Tina and were the main reason she decided to seek my help. Tina has studied hypnotherapy and understands that these visions may or may not be real events. She agrees that it doesn't matter to the mind whether they actually happened or are simply a creation of the psyche to explain her feelings about her sister. The fact was, they felt very real to her, and that was what mattered.

Tina shared that a few years earlier her mother had told her that Liz had always been jealous of her. Liz continues to have jealousy issues to this day. Tina's mother told her that she was very cute and outgoing as a child, while the older sister was sullen and shy. This outgoing, happy attitude caused Tina to get most of the attention of guests and family members and earned her the nickname Bubbles. Tina also had beautiful long white-blonde hair that caught the attention of almost everyone who saw her. Her older sister, on the other hand, had thin, wispy hair and was nearly bald until she was ten years old. When Tina was about five, her mother, exasperated by the older sister's jealousy, cut off Tina's beautiful hair, making it extremely short to match her sister's unattractive locks.

As they grew, Liz became obsessive about her body and her looks and was always dieting and exercising. Tina was involved in many other activities and paid little attention to her body until, as an older teen, she began gaining weight. As an adult, Tina admired and looked up to Liz and felt pride when cheering for her at her Liz's body building competitions. Tina, who was becoming more and more obese, also felt intense shame while attending these events, since they were so focused on looks and physique.

We began our EFT work with the statement:

Even though I am overweight, I deeply and completely love and accept myself.

In three rounds of tapping, her 0-to-10 intensity went from 10 to a 2. Tina yawned repeatedly during the tapping. We moved on.

Even though I have the memory of Liz pinching me…

Even though I have the memory of Liz smothering me with her hand…

Even though I have the memory of Liz smothering me with a pillow…

Even though Liz tried to kill me…

Even though my mother cut my hair to make Liz feel better about herself…

Even though Liz hates me…

Even though I hate Liz…

Even though I have to be diminished to make Liz feel OK…

Even though I have to be diminished or Liz will kill me…

Even though I have to stay fat to make Liz feel OK and not kill me…

Even though it is my fault that my son is fat…

The yawning continued, and Tina complained of being incredibly tired. She wanted to stop several times. However, we continued until there was no charge regarding thoughts of her sister.

Tina was obviously exhausted. She said she just couldn't do any more, then left and went straight to bed. She reported that she slept though the night and into the next day for a total of 13 hours of sleep.

The next day, she was stunned to find herself feeling relaxed and content. She had little or no emotional reaction to thoughts of her sister and resumed her weight loss plan with optimism and vigor. She has agreed to tap daily for any discomfort that may arise from thoughts of her sister and to tap for accepting a new, thinner self. She has released a lifetime of fear and pain regarding her sister and now has the tools and confidence to achieve her weight-loss goals.

❊ ❊ ❊

In this next report, Dr. Carol Solomon demonstrates how a core issue can affect us in more ways than one. This is a great illustration of not only how our emotional issues can be connected but also how while addressing one issue we can gain valuable insight into another. If you are ever stuck on an issue, you might try addressing another one for a while and see if any insights start to appear.

EFT for Panic Attacks and Overeating

by Dr. Carol Solomon

For ten years, my client Margie had panic attacks approximately twice a month in the middle of the night. She would wake up startled and feel "very, very scared...panicked...not knowing what to do." She had tightness in her chest and difficulty breathing. She felt as though she was going to jump out of her skin.

Margie's mother was depressed, very emotional, and easily overwhelmed. Everything was "hard" for her, and whenever something was hard, it threw her off. She couldn't handle it and became even more depressed.

Margie grew up telling herself that nothing was going to be hard for her and that she wouldn't make a big deal out of anything. Growing up, everything had been an issue, so Margie vowed not to let anything get to her. She thought that if she let anything get to her, it meant she was "weak," like her mom.

Margie sought my help to learn EFT for weight loss and overeating. Her way of getting things done was to eat her way through it. "I eat three cookies, and then I do the laundry."

Margie thought her panic attacks were triggered by feeling overwhelmed by problems. Even though she wanted everything to be easy, she was easily flustered and "thrown off" by unexpected events. She would overeat during the day to cope, but whenever she felt "too emotional," she had a panic attack at night. It was a terrifying experience.

Margie used to have to take medication to get back to sleep. Now, she starts tapping right away and it relieves the panicky feeling.

Even though I feel really scared right now, I deeply and completely accept myself.

Even though I feel alone and scared...

Even though I don't think I'll get through this...

Even though it feels like the morning will never come...

Even though I feel weak...

Even though I vowed that nothing would ever get to me, and I would always be strong...

Even though it's important to be stronger than my mother...

Then Reminder Phrases as she tapped around the body:

Feeling scared.

Feeling alone.

Can't breathe.

Feeling overwhelmed.

I don't know what to do.

It feels like the morning will never come.

I don't think I'll get through this.

I'm afraid I'll fall apart.

Since I had taught Margie EFT for weight loss, she included weight-related statements in her second round. Notice the similarity between feeling out of control and panicky with her life and feeling out of control with her food and weight-loss issues.

Even though I feel like my eating is out of control, I deeply and completely accept myself.

Even though I'm feeling fat…

Even though I'm not strong enough to deal with my problems…

Even though I feel like I'll never be strong enough and I'll always be overweight…

Even though I shouldn't have any issues with my body…

Then around the body:

Feeling scared.

Feeling fat.

I can't control my eating.

I'm not strong enough.

It's not OK to be weak.

I have to be strong all the time.

I shouldn't be having this anxiety attack.

I feel like I'm not going to make it.

Margie views EFT as a "fool-proof method" to short-circuit her panic attacks. It only takes one or two rounds for her to stop the panic attack and get back to sleep. She has had only one attack in the past four months and has not needed any medication. She has also significantly reduced her overeating.

❊ ❊ ❊

Most of the Setup language above was directed at global material rather than specific events. However, if you take a look at the last set of Reminder Phrases, from "feeling scared" to "I feel like I'm not going to make it," can you see how each one of those phrases could point to earlier events? What memories does she have that relate to feeling scared, being too weak, or being out of control?

If your issue is stubborn or you're having trouble getting to the core, try asking yourself similar questions based on the information you have already discovered.

In this next report, Cathleen Campbell describes a successful businesswoman who gained weight when her work conditions changed.

Her Boss Was Making Her Fat

by Cathleen Campbell

Joan came to me to work on a crisis that was brought on by a change in her career. She was thrilled to discover that in dealing with this issue we could also help her finally reach her health and fitness goals, too!

Joan is a lovely woman, full of enthusiasm and joy. She's had her ups and downs in life, but mostly she's lived a pretty wonderful life. Her career has always been a point of pride for her. She has worked in the same field for over two decades, accumulating an excellent salary and a wide assortment of awards and accolades.

One of the special joys Joan relied upon was the affectionate and supportive relationship she's always had with management, especially her immediate superior. She loved working with Beth because they not only had a tremendous respect for each other but they also just simply enjoyed each other's company.

Joan was both excited for her friend and nervous for herself when Beth accepted a new position, leaving the department and Joan behind. Joan wasn't sure she would be able to recreate the same relationship she cherished with another boss.

Weeks went by filled with trepidation and confusion. And then the bomb dropped. The new department manager was a woman who had been transferred many times, and rumor had it that she was both ineffective and disliked. Joan was about to live her worst nightmare.

Before long she was questioning her very career, let alone her job and her abilities. She was miserable. Each day was a horror. She would take sick days and find other ways to be out of the office as much as possible. By the time Joan started to work with me the situation had become critical. She was fearing the loss of her job and feeling as though she had the weight of the world around her shoulders…and her waist and thighs, etc.

We spent the first session clearing the pain she felt this new manager had inflicted, using specific incidents and wording such as:

Even though my new boss is so mean to me, she yelled at me yesterday in front of the whole department and I felt so ashamed especially since she was right, I deeply and completely accept myself.

Even though I'm nervous every time I talk to my new boss because she always seems so mad at me, I deeply and completely accept myself.

Even though I not only don't have the connection I've always relied on with my new boss, but it's worse than that since she apparently doesn't like me at all, I deeply and completely accept myself.

Since she hadn't known the new boss long, clearing this pain wasn't too difficult and Joan realized she was actually breathing easier and beginning to feel relaxed with this line of clearing. So we rolled up our sleeves and began to dismantle all the pain she had accumulated from the negative thoughts she'd been unable to stop thinking for months.

As we continued to clear through her personal criticisms, the ones she was aware of and the ones that she became conscious of as she continued to clear layer after layer, Joan began to sit up straighter and look more confidently assured. As if a light was slowly beginning to shine, dimly growing brighter with each layer lifted, Joan began to nod her head up and down. We finished a round and I asked her what she was nodding to, to which she replied, "I thought I was getting fat because of my age or the stress or my lack of exercise, but the truth is that I'm building a wall of protection around myself in every way I can!"

Joan's initial focus for her session work was her career, specifically clearing out the challenges with her new boss. She did this with very few tears and found it astonishingly easy. Now she was ready to face what was really getting her down: a load of added weight!

We began to tap for concepts such as:

Even though I have to protect myself from my boss in every way I can, which means I have to build myself up, I deeply and completely accept myself.

The look of relief on her face was a joy to behold, and her features began to appear calmer and younger. Joan left a bit exhausted but feeling terrific.

Over the next two weeks Joan kept in touch by email. Her final message said,

"I'm happy to report that I'm back to my usual habits—eating, drinking, exercise, sleeping, and performing at work. I feel happy and productive, and though my new boss is challenging, she's got some great ideas and we're started to get into a rhythm with each other. And the best news is that I've already dropped 10 pounds! It's melted off just as we said in session. My boss is not longer making me fat, but you know what? If she's right, she just might make my bank account a bit fatter!"

❉ ❉ ❉

The words of parents, teachers, coaches, partners, friends, and even total strangers can have a profound impact on our beliefs about ourselves. In this next report by Kathleen Sales, hurtful words held their sting for decades—until EFT removed their emotional impact. Her story is a great example of addressing a specific event for solid results.

Kathleen refers to the Sore Spot, which can be used in place of the Karate Chop point during the Setup Phrase, and the 9 Gamut Procedure, both of which are used in EFT's original Basic Recipe. They are not part of the EFT shortcut described in Chapter One, but they can be added at any time. See Appendix A for details.

"God, You're Fat!"
by Kathleen Sales

My client wanted to not only lose weight but also find a way to maintain that weight loss. She had tried many programs and had been successful at losing, but she always seemed to gain the weight back and then some.

I explained during our initial consultation that we could work on the issue of weight and maintenance but that we would also need to focus on emotional issues affecting her life since in most cases the issue of excess weight is not about the food at all. She agreed to the commitment and we were on our way.

I asked the typical questions about weight: *How long have you had a weight problem? When did you first recognize that you had a weight problem? Do others in your family struggle with weight?* And so on.

All of a sudden her face began to tense up as she spoke of her godmother, who had emotionally tortured her when she was young. Every weekend her family would make a trip to visit her godmother and godfather, and whenever no one was watching, Claire, her godmother, would exclaim, "God you're fat!" Keep in mind, this was said to a girl between the ages of six and seven, and it went on for three years.

The words echoing in her head brought great sadness and anger to the surface, so this is where we began. I asked her what her intensity rating was regarding this issue and she said, "Ohhhh, it's a 10 definitely!" While she massaged her Sore Spot, I had her close her eyes and repeat after me:

Even though I hear these cruel words, "God, you're fat," I deeply and completely love and accept myself.

Even though Claire's cruel words echo loudly, "God, you're fat," I deeply and completely accept myself and my body.

Even though I hear Claire's hurtful, mean, and cruel words, "God, you're fat," I completely love and accept myself anyway.

We then tapped on the EFT points using these Reminder Phrases:

> *God, you're fat!*
>
> *Those hateful cruel words, "God, you're fat."*
>
> *Claire's voice echoing, "God, you're fat."*
>
> *Those cruel hurtful words, "God, you're fat."*
>
> *God, you're fat!*
>
> *Claire's hateful, cruel voice saying, "God, you're fat."*
>
> *Claire's hurtful words, "God, you're fat."*
>
> *Those cruel, cruel words echoing inside of me, "God, you're fat."*

We also did the 9 Gamut Procedure, since this started at such a high intensity, followed by Setup Phrases to which we added the words *"this remaining…,"* and we did one last round of all the points while saying, *"I deeply and completely love and accept myself no matter what."*

I asked my client to remain with her eyes closed and go inside to see what was there. She felt a sense of calm. Her face had definitely relaxed, lightened up, and showed the results of the tapping. I then asked her to repeat the words, *"God you're fat!"* to see what, if anything, came up. She did and smiled. She said, "They're just words. They have no affect on me whatsoever. Claire is gone!"

At our next session I asked her to again repeat the words *"God you're fat!"* and absolutely nothing occurred. Just a smile and a shake of the head.

During the course of our work together, we found another person who needed to be "let go of," and when he surfaced my client said, "Oh goody, are we going to be able to make him disappear just like we did Claire?" We did, and it was another incredible result for EFT.

✿ ✿ ✿

Sneaking Up on the Core Issue

Sometimes the emotional reason for a craving or for overeating in general is an issue so overwhelming that it seems beyond help. It's the "Big One" that the person doesn't want to touch. It may be a major form of guilt that they don't want to face or a trauma they don't want to revisit. Whatever it is, they "don't want to go there" and often won't even mention it to their therapist for fear the therapist will try to drag them through it.

Often they learn to dull the pain or sweep it under the rug. But it seethes under the surface anyway, influencing their thoughts, their responses, and their everyday lives. It represents pain. It's like walking on thorns. They would rather retain their less-than-truly-functional lives than come face to face with this issue. Their lives will get better, they hope, if they just address life's minor irritations and leave the "Big One" alone.

Fortunately, we have a method with EFT whereby we can tip-toe up to the issue, circle around it, take the edge off, and gradually spiral in closer until that festering boil is skillfully lanced. All this with minimal pain. The concept is simple but it may take some practice before the practitioner can claim mastery.

It starts with a very general approach. I suggest asking the client simply say

The Big One

and then rank his or her 0-to-10 intensity regarding the mere mention of the issue. This is also an appropriate time to rank the intensity of other physical symptoms, such as a pounding heart, sweating, constricted throat, etc. We then use EFT in a general way to help take the edge off.

Even though I have discomfort about this issue, I deeply and completely accept myself.

Even though this thing seems too big for me…

Even though just thinking about it bothers me…

Even though my heart is pounding…

Even though [other physical symptoms]…

The details of the issue are ignored for now because the main purpose here is to minimize pain by taking the edge off. We are purposely sneaking up on the problem with gentleness as our goal. Do several rounds of EFT in this more general way until you see or experience signs of relaxation. That tell-tale "sigh" that I point out in our videotaped seminars is a good clue. Then say again…

The Big One

and re-rank the 0-to-10 intensities that this statement generates. Chances are the emotional responses will be lower and the physical symptoms will likely be down as well. I keep repeating this procedure until it seems appropriate to ask:

> *Is there any part of this issue that you could talk about comfortably?*

This simple procedure often opens the door, making it possible for the person to acknowledge or describe at least part of the issue. From there, it is simply a matter of getting more and more detailed. Take some of the edge off, get more detailed. Take some of the edge off, get more detailed. Take some of the edge off, get more detailed.

The client may experience some emotional discomfort in the process. After all, this *IS* the "Big One." But, in my experience, it is much less than it might have been *and* this is probably the last time the person will have any such discomfort. Assuming our usual degree of success, they can now walk on velvet instead of thorns.

❊ ❊ ❊

In this next report, Carol Look draws on her extensive experience with weight loss and addiction to provide valuable insights into common emotional drivers. Please note that this article provides many "doors" that you can use to explore your own issues. Once you find a good "door," you will still benefit from identifying the underlying specific events and releasing them with EFT.

A Compulsive Overeating and Weight-Loss Protocol

by Carol Look

Diets don't work because they cause people to feel deprived, which triggers emotional and behavioral "rebellion." Sooner or later, after feeling deprived, you will overeat to compensate for the feeling of deprivation. This means that if you are using a diet to curb your cravings, it will most likely backfire on you.

Diets don't work because starvation mode causes hormonal imbalances and when the body perceives the danger of starvation, it "hoards" calories and fat for safety. This is why so many people complain of gaining weight or staying at a plateau when they are certain that their caloric intake is insubstantial. They are right. Their caloric intake isn't enough for their bodies, yet they start to plateau or gain weight again.

Diets don't work because they focus on the wrong target—food—instead of the underlying emotions that cause people to overeat in the first place. If you are targeting food as the problem, you miss the underlying cause of overeating, which is emotional stress connected to your past, present, or future.

The Present

The first section of my EFT weight-loss protocol targets your current behavior or symptom. Obviously there are many layers under the symptom, but to attack these first is an easy way to get started. Also, some of the layers don't begin to emerge until you target eating behavior.

The primary phrases that clients give to me about their "addiction" or weight problem include:

Even though I'm a food addict, I deeply and completely accept myself.

Even though I'm obsessed with food…

Even though I'm a sugar addict…

Even though I crave sweets at night…

Even though I have an enormous appetite… (We'll get to the underlying cause of this "appetite" later.)

Even though I'm a closet eater…

Even though I binge at night…

I ask clients to tap for themselves three times a day for whichever of the above phrases speak to them and their problem. I ask them to do it in the early morning and late evening when they are not in the middle of a struggle to NOT eat. Those who wait until they have a craving are less likely to complete the process, although one can do it then as well.

Two more interesting phrases that really seem to help some clients are:

Even though I have an urge to eat whenever I SMELL food…"

Even though I have a craving whenever I SEE food…"

These are very powerful anchors. Remember, advertising works.

Then I move on to the underlying feelings and anxieties that drive the behavior. Classic phrases that hit home with clients include:

Even though I eat when I'm bored...
Even though I eat when I'm angry...
Even though I eat when I'm lonely...
Even though I overeat to hurt myself...
Even though I eat to avoid my feelings...
Even though I use food to soothe myself...
Even though I overeat to hide myself...
Even though I binge because I think I'm worthless...
Even though I overeat because I don't love myself...

I recommend that you go fishing for whatever phrases ring true. If you are working with a client, you will usually see it in the person's face or you will recognize when it hits home.

Two other key points that I find essential pertain to guilt and self-hatred. These are not motivating factors for people who want to lose weight, so I help them drop the guilt about their eating disorder.

Even though I hate myself for overeating...
Even though I feel guilty when I overeat...
Even though I feel guilty about being overweight...

It's important to reduce these feelings so they don't backfire and cause even more overeating as a result of the anxiety. I use the tapping point on the index finger and say, *"I forgive myself for overeating…or eating when I'm not hungry…or eating when I'm angry… etc.…."* This helps people forgive themselves for compulsive behavior that seems to be out of their control.

I worked for eight years at Freedom Institute with alcoholics, addicts, and their family members. The population termed ACOA deserves special mention. They are Adult Children of Alcoholics and were raised by one or more addicted parents or caregivers. "ACOAs" often suffer from free-floating guilt that would boggle your mind. They report feeling a gnawing sense of never being enough, never being a good enough child to help their parent stop drinking. *"If only I had been smart enough, good enough, clever enough, etc., mom would have stopped drinking for me."* Of course this isn't true, but eight-year-olds don't understand addiction. I always try to dig deep with clients who were raised with excessive dysfunction in order to get rid of the guilt and improve the chances of long-term success. Many ACOAs have sworn off alcohol because of their associations with an addicted parent but then turned to food as a more "acceptable" substance. Their underlying anxiety is often undiagnosed and untreated.

The Past

In this part of the treatment, I address basic self-esteem issues and incidents. I ask clients to write down or name three of the worst incidents that have hurt their self-esteem and tap for them. Often these incidents revolve around shame of their body or their early eating habits. I ask which is the loudest memory? The stickiest? The worst? I ask them to picture the first time they discovered food as a pacifier and address the underlying feelings that were going on at the time.

I also ask about their family's attitude about food, what the atmosphere was around the dinner table at home, etc. This often brings up new material, which I help them tap for.

Even though I'm anxious when I sit down to eat...

Even though I associate food with fighting...

Even though I associate food with my mother's love...

Even though I feel unsafe without food...

Even though I eat to feel better...

I ask clients to remember the sharpest criticism they heard around their body image, peer problems, etc. I have them tap for shame or whatever the strongest feelings are. This section can uncover upsetting times that may need more work. Go slowly and respectfully and you will make tremendous headway.

The Future

Next, I test clients to see how they would feel in the future if they couldn't binge with freedom. I ask them the following questions and tap for their reaction:

Picture yourself not being able to eat sweets in the evening. How do you feel?

They often say anxious, angry, lonely, or irritable. We tap for the response.

Picture yourself as thin as you would like. What happens? How do you feel?

This often brings up many answers. Sometimes they say they don't deserve it, or they feel anxious, or they don't feel safe anymore without their shield, etc. Sometimes they say they don't want other people to be envious of them or to comment on their body or appearance. We tap for whatever fears and feelings arise.

Picture yourself addressing the underlying feelings that trigger the eating behavior. How do you feel?

They often feel anxious or just "resistant" to doing it and admit that they would rather suffer with the eating and weight problems. Tapping might go something like this:

Even though I'm afraid to face my childhood depression...

Even though I'm afraid to deal with my rage at my father...

Then I address specific sabotaging behaviors and ask them what their theories are about why they might sabotage their progress. I ask them to say the following statements out loud and tap for whichever ones cause a reaction.

It's not safe for me to lose weight.

It's not safe for others if I lose weight.

I don't feel supported by my family members.

I have often heard about clients who are offered chocolate cake just as they are making progress in their weight-loss efforts.

I don't deserve to be happy with my body.

I ask them to say out loud, *"I weigh 125 pounds"* (or whatever their goal weight is) and see what emotions come up. As in some sports performance Setup Phrases that are highly effective, I have them tap say,

Even though I have a block about weighing less than 140 lbs...

Even though I sabotage myself whenever I weigh less than 130 lbs...

Even if I never get over this eating disorder...

Even if I never lose weight...

These last two seem to help the inevitable feelings of desperation that most people with binge-eating habits struggle with. The clients often say they don't want to say these phrases because they're not true. But I urge them to say them anyway. It seems to reduce unconscious energy blocks about losing weight and stopping out-of-control behavior.

Obviously there are many more phrases and issues you can tap for. It all depends on your particular patterns. The most universal problems that get in the way seem to be shame, guilt, self-hatred, and anxiety.

Extras

Apparently, restrictive eating, chronic dieting, yo-yo weight gain and loss, and basic binge eating disturb the balance of our endocrine system and thus the metabolism. This is particularly frustrating to clients who have thought that occasional starving in between binging can help them lose weight. The metabolism reacts by holding onto every last morsel of food, expecting to be starved again in the near future. This often slows down progress in the beginning for some people, as their metabolisms rebel by slowing down. This is why you often hear people say they don't eat enough food or calories to gain weight, yet they gain anyway. I ask my clients to read up on insulin production, the basics of nutrition, and how stress affects the hormonal system.

I know there is a lot of bad press about low-carbohydrate diets out there, but talk to a carbohydrate or sugar addict or someone who is hypoglycemic, and they will tell you that it does matter what kinds of foods they eat and when. They find that breads and sugars trigger a compulsion to eat more breads and sugars. This makes sense when you consider the basic principles of addiction. Alcoholics in Alcoholics

Anonymous (A.A.) know that "One drink is too many, and a million isn't enough." This is how a sugar addict feels about sugar. It can be effective to tap for:

> *Even though I'm out of control...*
>
> *Even though I'm powerless over food...*

Asking the Right Questions

It is essential to focus on the correct "target" for your EFT tapping session. I ask my clients key questions to uncover the emotions that are driving them to overeat.

> *What are you really starving for?*

We know that once you have satisfied your bodily needs for food, the remaining "hunger" is not physiologically driven, but driven by underlying anxiety or emotional conflict. See if you can identify what you may be starving for in your life, other than food.

What comfort was missing from your childhood? Love, affection, warmth, attention? This "absence" may be why you're overeating as an adult.

> *When do you experience cravings?*

It's important to identify the times of day when you feel vulnerable to giving in to your food cravings. Once you know your "weak" spots, you can apply EFT before these times, heading off your cravings before it's too late.

You may use EFT before these time frames, or during them, when you are actually experiencing a craving.

If you didn't eat something, what emotion would you feel?

If you weren't using food as a form of anesthesia, what emotions might surface for you? Sometimes people don't know the answer to this question because they've never been "without" the food. They continually overeat so the emotions don't surface — that's the point of the behavior. See if you can guess or intuit what the emotion of conflict might be if you didn't satisfy the craving. Then you will have a specific target for EFT.

When you don't have "enough" food, what feelings are you aware of? Irritability? Frustration? Panic?

Guidelines for Your EFT Sessions

Set aside 10 minutes twice or three times a day to take care of yourself and address the feelings that cause you to crave unhealthy foods and overeat. Some people prefer putting aside a longer period of time once a day. It doesn't matter as long as you make the commitment to yourself.

Make sure you can accomplish this commitment. If you need to make the time shorter when you get started, do so.

I recommend using a special notebook to record your feelings and insights from the questions you have asked yourself and from the answers you get from your tapping mini-sessions with yourself. Make notes about what surfaces during each session, and return to emotional conflicts or patterns that don't feel completed during your tapping session.

Be clear about your targets. Do you know exactly what you are tapping on?

Make sure you are tapping on *specific emotions* ("the guilt about…" "my anger towards…" "my hurt as a result of…") rather than global problems, such as "I have low self-esteem."

Make sure you are totally *tuned in to your emotions.* Turn off the television and other distractions like radios, cell phones, and telephone answering machines, and make sure you have set aside a safe space for yourself.

Be clear about your "before and after" measurements on the 0-to-10 point intensity scale. If you have assessed how high the anxiety is before you start tapping, you have a good "before" measurement to compare after your tapping session. Record your results.

Write down any "AHAs" that you get from your EFT sessions. You may use these insights for later tapping sessions.

Good luck and be persistent. You will notice that you will soon begin to "forget" about eating binges and instead plan your food. And you will become engaged in activities other than secretive eating or food shopping. The weight will begin to come off as the underlying issues are addressed and the basics of symptomatic behavior are tapped away.

❊ ❊ ❊

6

Eliminating Resistance

In any new project there are several ways in which we can interfere with our own progress. By becoming familiar with these ways, you can recognize them when they appear and then use EFT tapping to remove them.

By far the easiest way to reach a goal is with the cooperation of your subconscious mind. If there is agreement or congruence between what your conscious mind wants and what your subconscious mind has been programmed to accept as possible, everything is likely to flow smoothly toward the goal. But if there's disagreement or incongruence, the conscious mind doesn't have a chance. In that situation, the subconscious mind always wins. Somehow circumstances will conspire to prevent you from reaching your goal, and the conscious mind will probably never understand what happened or why. It will simply forget about the project or attribute your failure to bad luck or circumstances. It won't know that you yourself went out of your way to prevent your own success.

If you have ever made a New Year's resolution regarding your weight or physical fitness, you understand this syndrome all too well. Your conscious mind really wants to get your body into shape, and you may even start your new diet and exercise program with enthusiasm. But a week later, you're back on the sofa watching TV and eating potato chips.

Resistance to improving your life can show up in several forms. We have already discussed Psychological Reversal and tail-enders, both of which tend to operate behind the scenes and can be difficult to see. In this chapter, we'll look at more obvious, conscious forms of resistance and some easy ways to address them.

EFT can be effective even if you don't believe it will work and even if part of you doesn't want it to. Irene Mitchell, who learned EFT while recovering from a car accident, discovered this two years ago. She explains:

> In March, my daughter invited me to go on a cruise with her. She said that I had to lose at least ten pounds, though, as one gains a lot of weight on a week-long cruise. I had never practiced EFT for weight loss before, but I decided to try it. I kept at it and tapped every time I wanted to eat things I shouldn't. Sometimes I had to tap for the desire to tap.

> *Even though I don't want to tap about this weight problem because I really want to eat whatever I want...*

> After two months of tapping all the time and following a balanced diet, I dropped 25 pounds!! I have *never* had such a dramatic weight loss, ever!! Aside from the weight loss, there were unexpected benefits.

Naturally, I could get around better. I had less pain in my injured leg (which makes sense when you are lugging around less weight) and navigating in the shower was a lot easier. The best, though, was the fact that my sugar readings went so low that I had to go from 25 units of insulin each night to only five! My doctor is thrilled! So am I!

❊ ❊ ❊

Go to the health section of any major book store and you will find several books pointing the finger at sugar as the villain behind many of our physical ailments. Like tobacco and alcohol, sugar saps away our mental and physical functioning in insidious ways. Also like tobacco and alcohol, sugar can be an addictive substance. This contributes, of course, to a downward spiral wherein we crave more and more of that which is soaking up our vitality.

Helen Powell has faced a lifetime of sugar consumption and addiction, and she recently used tapping to clear herself of the problem. Please note the emphatic way in which she applied the process one evening. She says, *"I said it vehemently, I yelled it out, I listened to every word, I felt my resistance..."* This approach is often effective for stubborn issues. Here is Helen's story.

Emphatic Tapping for a Sugar Addiction
by Helen Powell

I too have a story to add to the countless amazing stories that abound in the world of EFT. Last

November I realized I simply *had to give up* the huge quantities of chocolate and ice cream that I was eating several times a week and sometimes daily. About ten years ago I began to notice a decline in my mental functioning and eyesight. I've read enough to know that it could be the sugar that was addling my mind but I just felt powerless before these strong cravings. Since then I began to experience more and more confusion, high levels of stress, difficulty in making decisions, mental fatigue, and more fears. Thank goodness, I don't have diabetes.

I took my first tapping course about four years ago. Since then I have used EFT with my clients and know how marvelously effective it can be. Even so, I wondered if tapping on this problem would *really* help *me*. The bottom line in truth was that I didn't want to tap away my fix. However, last summer and fall I did something so bizarre that I got scared. In October I did two brief tappings on *"I eat too much sugar"* but nothing happened, probably because my heart was not really in it. But maybe even that minimal tapping helped prepare the way because one November night, in desperation, I faced my strong reluctance to give up this bad behavior.

I started with the Karate Chop point, tapping on:

I don't want to stop eating all the ice cream and chocolate I eat, I just don't want to give it up, and I accept and forgive myself anyway.

I said it vehemently, I yelled it out, I listened to every word, I felt my resistance and accepted that this is just the way it is for now. I became fully engaged in the process. I did several rounds without bothering to measure my intensity on the 0-to-10 scale and then went to bed.

That was five months ago. Since that night, I have refused all desserts. What is interesting to me is when I look at all those "goodies" (are they really "good"?) something in me just holds back and refuses even though I can almost taste them. I have never felt deprived, not even for a moment. I've been to a couple of birthday parties where I surprisingly ate a piece of birthday cake without thinking, but I haven't accepted any other dessert without thinking as I was wont to do in the past. Maybe it was OK for me to do that because cake has never been my sweet of choice. I never felt guilty or frightened by these two isolated acts.

In January, I tested myself after looking longingly at a small package of jelly beans (no chocolate). I did buy it, and they did taste good, but I didn't really enjoy them. I don't consider any of those events lapses. And I am very happy to say I no longer feel as if I am losing my mind. The persistent haze that clouded my eyesight has disappeared as well. I feel much more confident and again really positive about myself and my future. Let me also add that I am 77 years old looking back at a lifetime of chocolate and ice cream abuse.

❋ ❋ ❋

Here's a useful perspective by Angela Treat Lyon which points to emotional aspects that could underlie the stubbornness of some weight issues.

A Unique Perspective on Weight Loss
by Angela Treat Lyon

I've been working with an acupuncturist who uses Traditional Chinese Medicinal Herbs to help me drain the edema I have experienced since I was a young teenager. For years I had simply thought, "I'm fat. I'm overweight."

I had tried every last thing on the planet to resolve this weight imbalance and was at my last wit's end. I had dropped about 30 pounds already with what I thought was better eating and exercise. I had used EFT to overcome a chocolate/white sugar addiction—which worked like a dream the very first time, and I haven't even wanted chocolate since—and this is from someone who was practically weaned on chocolate. No more candy. What a relief!

Still, I needed to drop another 20 pounds before feeling close to my "natural" weight, where I'd feel light and strong and have energy without strain on my heart or muscles. I'd been carrying around the extra weight for so long that I had to buy bigger shoes, and I had been wearing men's extra-large shirts just to cover my large bottom. This all even after the great strides I had made since learning about EFT!

The acupuncturist told me that some of what I had been doing only exacerbated the problem. She said I was to avoid cold foods (no yogurt? no protein shakes?) because their damp condition made my whole body swell up. I love cold food. I was bummed. And she told me that my heart was weakened and very tired and that I needed to tone down my workouts to reduce my heart rate. I like to work out hard. Feels good. I was bummed again. And scared—my heart is *weak?* And *tired?*

I did a mini-rebellion and took the herbs she prescribed—but I ate the cold things anyway. And worked out just as hard.

And felt more tired, and more groggy, and more mentally inept and foggy. After a few days of this, I had to really ask myself, What am I doing? I'm paying to see her, yet I'm not doing what she recommends. So I asked myself why I would rebel against someone to whom I had gone for help. It was like saying, "No, no, don't help me down the ladder when my house is burning!" Duh!

So I tapped on:

Even though I hate it that she programmed me to think of my heart as weak and tired, I deeply and completely accept myself.

Even though I hate it that I have to cook more…

Even though I hate it that I can't eat my favorite foods and I hate it that someone is telling me what to do…

Even though she programmed me...

Even though it's all her fault...

Even though I think I have to cook more and it takes too much time...

Even though I have to eat food I really don't want...

Even though I have to do what she says...

...I deeply and completely love and accept myself, and I forgive myself and anyone else for my having gotten here in the first place.

I looked deeper. Thinking that my more-than-40-year-old problem was her fault was absurd to the extreme – she wasn't even born when it started! I felt as if no matter what I did, it was wrong: that I broke out or got sleepy or became anxious or had some kind of unpleasant symptom no matter what I ate, and I'd rather not eat than go through all this. I'd rather die than hassle all this. I wondered—was I psychologically reversed to *living?*

So I tapped:

Even though it's not my fault...

Even though I want to blame someone else —anyone else —for my problems...

Even though I'd rather die than have to go through all this...

Even though I want to die, I don't want to be here...

Even though I'll never get it right...

Even though this is too much trouble...

Even though all food is bad for me...

Even though I can't eat anything or have any sat-
isfaction...

...I deeply and completely love and accept myself.

I can't have any satisfaction? Whew! That hit
deep. I looked at how I had made a career out of
being creative and resourceful, and how I flew from
one project to the next without giving myself room for
congratulations or celebrating what I had just accomplished. Why on earth not?

So I tapped on:

Even though I am never satisfied...

Even though I have no real idea what that would
feel like...

Even though I don't give myself the credit I deserve...

...I deeply and completely love and accept myself
and everything I do or accomplish, and I choose to stop
and congratulate myself and celebrate from now on, even
if it's for only a moment, and I'll grow it more and more
each time, because I deserve it.

I have been tapping on all those thing for four or
five days.

Today I noticed a pronounced difference in my
body. My pants are slipping off my hips (!!!) and I
feel not just slimmer but more compact somehow. I
can see it in the mirror, too.

I am now even more firmly convinced that it's not *only* food that goes in and out of our bodies, and it's not only what kind of or how much exercise we get. We also need to manage the energy in our body-mind system.

❊ ❊ ❊

When all else fails, persistence with EFT is usually the answer. Virginia Sabedra and her sister created a personal "EFT marathon" for weight loss while driving for an hour and a half in a car. The tapping led them from tail-ender to tail-ender on a journey that revealed many "behind the scenes" issues. To me, overweight is never a problem in and of itself. Rather, it is a *symptom* of other issues, many of them hidden. Personal EFT marathons may be a great way to bring them out.

Personal EFT Marathon

by Virginia Sabedra

Thought I'd share an experience I had a few weeks ago with EFT and my sister. My sister came to town to visit me. Since I had planned on taking a "fun" class in Oakland (which is 98 miles from Sacramento, where I live), I asked my sister if she'd like to take the class as well. She jumped at the chance and on Saturday morning, we got up early, got in the car, and headed for Oakland.

As soon as we were on the freeway, I told my sister that I was concerned about some weight I was gaining and asked if she would like to work on this with me. She said she'd love to because this is an area she would like to work on as well.

She was a little familiar with EFT from my visit to her home a year ago. When I arrived at her house back then, she couldn't move her arm without pain. The first thing I asked her was, "What is it that you are shouldering?"

She laughed and then I guided her through EFT for about 20 minutes as her pain and stiffness melted away.

Anyway, back to the car and driving to Oakland. The drive is about one and a half hours long. We began EFT with the first thought about weight that popped into our minds, then that brought up another and another. Thoughts, beliefs, feeling, and ideas about weight and food abounded.

This belief that food is bad...

This belief that all I have to do is walk past a bakery and I gain weight...

This belief that the older we get the wider we get...

This fear that I'll never be slim and trim...

Tail-ender after tail-ender. We discovered that even the tail-enders have tail-enders.

After ninety minutes of tapping, laughter, sadness, surprises, and revelations, we arrived in Oakland and headed for our class. We wondered what the people in other cars passing us by had thought about us, two women in a car tapping their faces and upper bodies while mouthing words. We concluded that pretty soon tapping in cars will be a familiar sight. By the way, I was driving very carefully.

After our most excellent class we headed for San Francisco to have dinner. Then we headed home for another hour and a half of EFT and weight. You will not believe the "stuff" that came up with us both working on the same issue. When one of us came up with a super-meaningful tail-ender, we'd encourage one another with *"Ahhh, that's a good one,"* or *"Oooooh, that hits home for me,"* and so on as we just continued on and on, tapping, releasing and releasing and tapping, both of us throwing things into the pot, all the gunk about weight, food, women, traditions, holding on, getting your money's worth, etc. It was an amazing, eye-opening, revelation-inducing process about all the stuff we had stuffed ourselves with, as well as all the stuff that we allowed to be stuffed into us.

The next day, both my sister and I commented on how our San Francisco dinner had been different somehow. We thoroughly enjoyed our food, yet it was different. There was a freedom or lack of any thought about fat, fear, calories, and so on. Yet, we were observant of the food. It had a presence to it. We loved the food and how it was prepared. We ate differently in mind and body. I can't explain it well except to say that a shift of some sort had taken place.

The next day my sister's visit ended and she left. About four days later, I called my sister and asked if she had noticed anything about going to the bathroom. She stated that now that I had mentioned it, yes. She hasn't been constipated. I reported the same thing. Since our marathon, I have been regular. I mean nice and regular. I had always had a problem with this. My sister has always had a problem also. Yet, we both reported a cessation of constipation since our EFT marathon. Was it weight-related? In this case, I'd say so.

My sister and I are planning a second marathon on the same subject to see what else comes up and what results we will get, or where it will lead. We realize we have years upon years, and generations upon generations, of worn out, old, outdated beliefs, ideas, feelings, and notions to release.

I would say that during our marathon, we released months, perhaps years, worth of work on the subject of falseness, illusions, and negativity around weight and food, and other related subjects that automatically came up. In fact, I'm still processing to this day.

I have stopped gaining weight. Constipation-wise, I am *"nice and easy"* now. I spontaneously bless the food I eat. I ask and expect my body to process the food I eat and to let go of all that I don't need in a healthy way, and I am learning to appreciate myself in many ways.

I know that I am not "done" yet with my work. And, this is OK because as we work we continue to seek, explore, savor, experience, learn, appreciate, heal, and live.

This experience gave me the idea to conduct EFT marathons on various subjects. I conducted an EFT marathon on the subject of money in my office with a small group and it went very well. The collective consciousness of two or more people working and tapping on the same problem or subject has proven to be powerful.

❈ ❈ ❈

7

Eating Disorders

EFT can do more than help the overweight lose pounds and inches. It can help those with eating disorders improve their health and develop a more normal relationship with food.

Of the many eating disorders that occur in humans, two of the most widely known are anorexia nervosa and bulimia.

Anorexia, a condition in which people starve themselves, can occur in men and women of any age, but it is most associated with adolescent girls. By itself, the term *anorexia* refers to a loss of appetite, while *anorexia nervosa* describes a psychological disorder.

Anorexia nervosa's most obvious symptom is extreme thinness, a body weight at least 15 percent below normal. Despite their thinness, those who suffer from anorexia nervosa have a distorted body image and see themselves as overweight. Three common ways in which they prevent weight gain are with excessive exercise, the use of laxatives, and by avoiding food.

A binge is any behavior indulged to excess, such as drinking, gambling, eating, or spending. Binge eating or bingeing refers to the practice of eating until one is beyond full. People who binge seldom notice what they are eating or how it tastes. This type of compulsive out-of-control eating is very different from the experience of appreciating, savoring, and enjoying one's food.

Bulimia, a binge-and-purge disorder, involves eating large amounts of food and then vomiting to remove it. An out-of-control appetite, feelings of anger and frustration, a history of fasting, the frequent use of enemas, purgative laxatives, or diuretics, and compulsive exercise may be additional factors. Often dentists are the first medical professionals to notice or diagnose bulimia because it harms tooth enamel and damages the esophagus. Bulimia also harms the stomach, can lead to dangerous metabolic imbalances, contributes to heart problems, and seriously interferes with the assimilation of nutrients, leading to malnutrition.

It has long been my view that anorexia, binge eating, and bulimia are not problems in and of themselves. Neither are addictions, cancer, and a long list of other ailments and behaviors. Rather, these are often *symptoms* caused by unresolved anger, guilt, fear, and other harmful emotions that cause conflicts (lack of peace) within the system. Until they are properly resolved, we may just flit from symptom to symptom with the illusion that healing is taking place.

We do the best we can given our existing beliefs, attitudes, and other resources. But now we have a new understanding of what healing is about. Our new energy-based techniques are *shouting* at us to re-evaluate our previous procedures. With their use, such things as head-aches, stomach distress, depression, orthopedic problems, and lactose intolerance have gone completely away without pills or surgeries. Even the most intense emotional issues have often subsided without a trace of their return.

Until now, bulimia and other forms of eating disorders have rarely been cured. Rather, they have been treated by a variety of means in hopes they would "get better."

But EFT is changing that outcome. As practitioners around the world are discovering, tapping while focusing on the underlying causes of eating disorders can completely change a person's self-image, relationship with food, physical appearance, and overall health.

Keep in mind that conditions like anorexia and bulimia are very serious and have been considered life-threatening. Accordingly, approaching an eating disorder with EFT should be done with significant caution, solid experience, and often with the advice of a physician.

In this chapter, we will explore some individual cases related to eating disorders so you can see the complexity of emotional issues that we often find underneath them. You will also see how experienced EFT professionals have used their creativity and experience to work through them.

Unlike the other chapters, this information is not intended as instruction for using EFT to "cure" an eating disorder. Rather, it is provided as introductory information for anyone who is considering EFT as an addition to their treatment program. If you have been diagnosed with an eating disorder, please enlist the help of an experienced EFT Practitioner and consult with your physician before you add EFT to your treatment program.

Now that we have the proper precautions out of the way, let's move on to some real life cases.

Karl Dawson of the U.K. walks us through the intricacies of a successful anorexia case in this entertaining story. As you will see, there were many related aspects and core issues that had to be handled before the client, Joe, could resume eating normally.

Joe Resolves His Anorexia—and More

by Karl Dawson

At the time I was working with this client, there was very little on the EFT website regarding anorexia. I hope this article may help other practitioners tackle this issue. I did feel at the time that it was a borderline case and I was in danger of going "where I didn't belong." But, after speaking to Joe, I knew he had given up on the health care professionals. And as far as his parents were concerned, "the professionals" had given up on Joe. So I knew I had to try.

Joe's main problem was anorexia, having gone from 13 stone (182 pounds or 82.5 kilograms) to 8 stone (112 pounds or 51 kilograms) over a nine-month period, compounded by extreme anxiety, panic attacks, and self-harming behavior. Other issues that became apparent were an addiction to the artificial sweetener Aspartame, Attention Deficit Disorder, and feeling a loss of control in life.

Treatment consisted of eight two-hour sessions over a period of four weeks. Four of the sessions occurred in the final week of treatment, after Joe had been sent home from work because he passed out and was told to remain off work until his problems had been "dealt with."

In the first session I concentrated on gaining Joe's trust and mapping out some of the core issues that led a highly intelligent teenager from a good loving home to develop all of these problems. Joe insisted that his girlfriend sit in on this first session. This concerned me at first, but Emma was very helpful in encouraging Joe to work with me and happily tapped along, putting Joe at ease.

One of the first glaring issues was Joe's (and Emma's) addiction to Diet Coke, which is sweetened with Aspartame, a controversial calorie-free artificial sweetener which some regard as highly addictive neurotoxin that is added to many diet products. Joe consumed up to 15 cans of Diet Coke a day in order to suppress his appetite and maintain a daily calorie intake below 500 calories.

We all tapped on this addiction issue with simple Setup Phrases:

Even though I have this addiction to Diet Coke, I deeply and completely accept myself.

Even though this Coke helps me suppress my appetite...

Even though I'm afraid I will eat more if I don't drink lots of Diet Coke...

Even though I'll feel hungry if I stop drinking lots of Diet Coke...

Very quickly Joe reported a loss of interest in Coke and his consumption dramatically decreased over the next few days to the occasional can and then to zero.

This first success was critical in my view because it gave a quick positive example of the effectiveness of EFT, giving Joe belief in the process, and it also got him off Diet Coke/Aspartame, which turned out to be one of the triggers behind his panic attacks.

The following events happened around the time of our first few sessions and illustrate Joe's frame of mind at the time.

Joe's parents had hidden the scales in order to stop him obsessing about his weight. Joe found the scales and weighed himself just as his dad entered the room. Seeing that his weight had gone up a few pounds, in conjunction with his dad observing this (In Joe's mind he was letting his parents down again in the only area of control he had in life), sent Joe into a suicidal panic. Joe disappeared for a few hours and returned with cuts and grazes to his hands and face. When I spoke with him later, he was in a desperate state and just wanted to give up. "I'm sick of trying," he said, "I don't care anymore."

I got a call early one Saturday morning from Joe's mother asking if I could come round. Something had happened that I never got to the bottom of, but when I met Joe at his house, he was in a highly distressed state. For 15 minutes or so I just tapped through the EFT points, occasionally repeating, *"This emotion, this anxiety, this panic.'* Joe eventually calmed down but was not in the mood to carry on with a session.

After talking to his parents for five minutes, I went to check on Joe before leaving. Joe was having his hair cut by Emma and was perfectly calm. Joe recently told me that earlier that day he had been *"only a slight breeze away from ending up in front of a train."*

The dilemma was the eating issue. The last thing anorexics want to talk about or adjust is their food intake, but unless we consume at least 800 calories per day, the brain is starved of nutrition making any logical thinking difficult.

Joe had also grown wary of health professionals. He had already been treated by his General Practitioner, crisis team, psychologist, and anorexic specialists, all of whom he felt had abandoned him and let him down. Joe was under the impression that they were waiting for his weight to fall a little lower so they could hospitalize and force-feed him.

Knowing that staying away from the food issue was the only way forward, we talked about other things that were bothering him. I used Gary Craig's favorite question:

If there was an event in your life you wish had never happened, what would it be?

It very quickly became apparent that a lot of Joe's problems had started around the age of six or seven at school. Until then he'd been a happy, carefree child. This I confirmed in a telephone conversation with his mother.

Joe's teacher that year was an elderly, old-school disciplinarian. From talking to Joe it was obvious he'd had some degree of Attention Deficit Disorder and/or Dyslexia, which had never been diagnosed. At the same time he was obviously very intelligent, leaving the teacher to draw the wrong conclusions.

In the first sessions Joe's memory of these events was vague to non-existent. In my subsequent talk with Joe's mother, she provided me with small amounts information, and we began to piece events together, sometimes just guessing what the teacher might have said in these situations.

The more we tapped, the more Joe remembered. Slowly at first, he started to recall memories which eventually flooded out, to the point were I had to write quickly to keep track on these issues to work on later.

I will let some of the Setup Phrases we used over the sessions tell the story of what had transpired between Joe and his teacher that year.

Even though I found it hard to concentrate...

Even though I found it hard to do math...

Even though I had trouble reading...

Even though I didn't pay attention to the teacher...

Even though Mrs. Smith said I was stupid...

Even though she said I was a little monster...

Even though I felt out of control...

Even though I would panic and shout out silly answers...

Even though nobody wanted to be my friend...

Even though I was different from the other kids...

Even tough I had to sit on my own away from other kids...

Even though the other kids laughed at me...

Even though I didn't fit in...

Even though my parents were called to school...

Even though the teacher told my parents I'm bad...

Even though my parents believed everything the teacher said...

Even though she said she tried to make me cry to get some emotion from me...

Even though my parents were angry with me for not trying...

Even though the harder I tried the worse I did...

Even though I let my parents down...

Even though I had terrible headaches…

Even though I gave up trying…

There were also many mental movies we had to work through, each one having several intense emotional highs and many aspects. A brief description of these were;

One day Joe found a note in his desk and on it was a list of things he had done wrong. His teacher said it had been left there by mistake, but Joe was terrified his parents would get to see it.

In her "infinite wisdom," the teacher thought tying Joe to his desk would be an excellent way to stop him fidgeting.

Joe had seen one of the other children dotting ink on his hands. He told a few of the other kids that the boy had measles. When the teacher heard Joe, she made a huge deal out of it and took the kid with the spots out of the class, telling them she was going to call the doctor and the boy's parents. Joe was left shocked and afraid of the consequences of his joke.

One day Joe and his brothers were being picked up from school. In a rush Joe's mum handed him a check and told him to hold it. Joe absent-mindedly put it in his pocket. His mother forgot she gave it to him and frantically looked for it for days. He did not remember having it until he found it in his pocket at school a few days later. He again felt he had let his parents down and was afraid to tell them, as they might think he had been bad again.

We also tapped using the Movie Technique on several recurrent nightmares he'd had at that age. He hated night-time, due to intense headaches and the fear of these nightmares.

In the main dream, he was alone inside his house and there was something dark and threatening trying to get inside the house and attack his sleeping family. (It struck me that these repeated dreams would also likely be trapped in his energy system. Would his subconscious have been able to differentiate between these nightmares and reality?)

It took a lot of tapping and reframing to bring the intensity of these dreams down. Again, at the start his memory was sketchy, but as we cleared one area, a new part of the dream would open up, and they were indeed scary.

Eventually Joe was able to go through the whole nightmare without emotion. He even gave his understanding on the dreams meaning. The exact understanding escapes me, but it had something to do with being petrified of having no control over events in his life and the effect his behavior had on his family.

Around this time in the EFT newsletter there was an article by Rebecca Marina describing the "Volcano Technique," in which clients are encouraged to feel and express their anger about situations that upset them. Because Joe often experienced extreme anger, we used this technique several times. As described in the article, anger can be a very empowering emotion. Giving clients license to really vent their anger — while tapping—helps to bring out and explode many other emotions. I found this method very powerful and have used it many times since.

Joe at 18 is a very polite, well-mannered young man. Even so, I think some of the language he used while we experimented with the volcano technique can be left to the imagination.

By our seventh session, Joe was ready to forgive his teacher, putting the way he was treated down to a misunderstanding on her part. He was also willing to forgive himself!

We did our last session over the phone. It was our fourth session that week, Joe had been very brave and had put a lot of effort into the sessions and was also doing a lot of tapping on his own. This was critical, especially with Joe. Self-empowerment of clients to me is one of the key elements and benefits of EFT.

It was our first and only telephone session. Something was on Joe's mind this evening, but he would not say exactly what it was. Joe had cleared an incredible amount of personal baggage, having undergone huge cognitive changes, in the process regaining a lot of self-respect and much more personal freedom.

In retrospect, I realize Joe was toying with the idea of seeing if he was capable of relinquishing his need to control his eating as his only form of control in life. Metaphorically I had a sense Joe was trying to reach the pivotal point of a seesaw. If he could find the faith to get past this point, his struggle would be an easy downhill ride—but he would have to let go and trust himself. We talked and tapped for an hour and he said he felt better. We set up an appointment for the next day.

Joe called me early the next morning, saying that he had decided to start eating again and that he wanted to cancel the appointment. Although obviously pleased, I was also concerned. That weekend I kept in contact with Joe's parents, and they confirmed he had started eating properly. Like me, they were cautiously optimistic.

Two weeks later Joe returned to work. He called me a few days before returning, saying he was slightly worried about facing the people at work, scared that the pressure and the attention he would get from them might be too much for him. He said he would tap on it.

A few days after he called to say he had gone to McDonald's with everyone from work to prove that he was OK now. But he gave the Diet Coke a miss.

I spoke with Joe this week for the first time in over four months. He now weighs 12 stone (168 pounds or 76 kilograms), is happy with his weight, and could never imagine so much as going on a diet. At the same time, he is worried he eats a little to much "crap food."

I wanted to ask him if it was OK to write this case study. He said, *"I believe your help and EFT saved my life. If it can help others, please write anything you want."* He said he is still tapping—when he needs it. At times he feels a little compulsive, such as when he feels under pressure, but EFT always helps.

He and Emma are saving up, as they want to travel round the world next year. He said he still thinks about what happened to him earlier that year and it scares him when he does. But now he says he feels 130 percent confident most of the time and can't believe how things got so out of control. "It seems like it happened to someone else," he says. He says he wishes he could get his mum and dad to do some tapping. *"It's about time they started dealing with some of their issues!"*

✻ ✻ ✻

We all overeat from time to time, especially at Thanksgiving and other holidays. In social situations that encourage overeating, it's hard to resist a second or third helping or another dessert. But when overeating occurs frequently and becomes a cause of shame or embarrassment, or when it becomes a darkly guarded secret, it moves from being an occasional indulgence to being a compulsion, a psychological disorder over which you have no control.

Binge eating has many emotional roots, many of which are often outside the person's conscious awareness. In this report, Dr. Carol Solomon shares her process with Carla's binge eating, then Carla shares her experience with food as a result of those sessions.

EFT Success for a Binge Eater

by Dr. Carol Solomon

To a binge eater, having one experience where you feel comfortable in your own skin is a success. Throwing away food because you didn't want it is a major breakthrough. A day without bingeing can feel like a miracle.

I have worked with Carla for four sessions. She had a traumatic childhood because of an abusive father. She associated food with survival, the only thing she could give herself for comfort. As a child, she promised herself that when she grew up, she could have whatever she wanted, whenever she wanted.

Carla already knew that EFT worked, since she used it to eliminate her need for her asthma inhaler. But she had not been able to stop binge eating. This problem can permeate everything you do. Carla had her life on hold. She wanted to build her business and start a new relationship, but everything felt too risky. The world was not a safe place.

First, we tapped on her belief that she can't have what she wants, so she substitutes food.

Then we tapped on her fear of promoting herself, of making mistakes, of the consequences of those mistakes, and her fear of being judged.

Finally, we tapped on one specific traumatic event, her sense of feeling unsafe in the world, and using food to ward off feelings of emptiness.

Here is Carla's letter to me:

Hi there Carol—Just wanted to update you that I seem to have had a breakthrough with our last session, although elements of earlier sessions are now accessible all at the same time!

Have not binged since Saturday's call without white knuckling (!!!!!) and I have in fact been having three regular (full of real food, but not grotesque quantities—just regular sized full of variety) meals!!!

For the first time in my *life* I threw chocolate away. On Monday night, I was given a chocolate at the end of Christmas meal with friends at a restaurant and I put it to my mouth to take a bite (habit—it was in my mouth before I thought about it) and it was too sweet and I was too full …and I held the last two-thirds of it in my fingers for over 10 minutes as we were all saying goodbye, and I threw it in a bin *(threw it out)* on the way to my car!!!

I watched all the team at work pig out on candy-colored donuts at 9:30 a.m. and couldn't imagine anything worse so joined them without eating, without feeling like I cared what they thought (and they didn't!), and I was totally comfortable with it—*comfortable!*

I have re-tapped to Saturday's recording several times. I have also been tapping on more words around the language you have given me, such as, "That was then, this is now," which is really powerful. Lots of tapping with words coming to me easily around the promise I made to myself that was so strong through my childhood—my daily survival mantra—that when I grew up I could have whatever I wanted, whenever I wanted it. I really believed to my emotional core that food was the path, and only path, to my happiness.

It has "clicked" in me that actually that was then, and it was a little muddled, albeit well intentioned, and I can still honor my promise, just in a way that leads to my happiness by allowing me to be open to the things I want.

The tapping also seems to have kind of wired me up to comfortably connect with the new thought that salad and fish or salad and steak (*salad* and *meat* and *no dessert*—what is going on?) is actually the path to my happiness. I have always been able to physically feel better eating regular sized meals and easily digestible foods but my emotional drive to eat fast food fast, and lots of it, has always outweighed my physical discomfort every time.

These last few days feel profoundly different to me. My words to you are not sufficient for explaining right now—but they will give you an idea of how I feel so different!

I am nervous it won't last, so am tapping on that too. But that is the point, I am tapping (not refusing to tap), allowing myself to buy and prepare food, go to bed on time, and do the things that I want to do rather than assume it is too hard or scary and cop out and eat instead.

Today, I have the energy that comes from not being fueled only by junk food—amazing—so in itself, it is a relief.

It is unbelievably exciting—because I am not "trying." Today is Thursday, we spoke Saturday, and it has sort of just happened. It also feels like I have had a "click" in that I have been allowing myself to distract myself from the habit of constantly calculating the calorie restrictions needed for 40 kilos to come off in just a few weeks so that I magically get thin fast. I am feeling I can focus on just living and for three days have had no problem with taking time off from work or activity to have a proper meal. No Coca Cola in sight.

And on and on I could go…Much love and appreciation,

Carla

As practitioners, we have this driving need to help people, and it's easy to forget how much difference we can make in people's lives and in the world. When I receive letters like this from clients, I remember, and I am grateful for EFT and all of the wonderful practitioners who have dedicated their lives to helping others.

❖ ❖ ❖

After that letter from Carla, we might assume that four sessions was enough to tackle her binge eating. However, as Carol and Carla kept working, deeper issues continued to surface. The following is a second report of Carla's journey after eight more sessions. Listen in as Dr. Solomon helps discover, and resolve, several core issues.

Binge Eating Recovery

by Dr. Carol Solomon

My client, Carla, was aching to stop binge eating so that she could become more slender. As much as she wanted to lose weight, Carla viewed thin people as vulnerable, exposed, and weak. She somehow feared that she would "blow away in the wind" if she became thin. She thought she was being "shallow" in her beliefs about thin people, but it turned out to be much deeper than that and, as we worked, several core emotional issues emerged.

Even though I think thin people are weak, and I don't want to be like them, I love and accept myself completely.

Even though I'm afraid I'll blow away in the wind if I don't eat enough...

Even though I think thin people are exposed and vulnerable...

Even though I'm not sure what this means, or how I came to believe this...it feels threatening...like I might not even exist if I don't eat enough.

Reminder Phrases:

Thin people are weak.

Thin people are vulnerable.

Thin people are exposed.

They can't protect themselves.

I don't want to be like them.

I might blow away in the wind.

It doesn't feel safe to lose weight.

I don't know what this means, but it feels like some scary times I had in my past...like my very existence was threatened.

Through this sequence, Carla made some important connections. As a child, Carla's parents made her eat three meals per day, so that she wouldn't get "too thin," but restricted her from eating junk food.

Carla often felt deprived, so she would binge-eat in secret, and then eat her meals anyway, so her parents wouldn't suspect that she was bingeing. Whatever she was deprived of...that's what she craved. As an adult, Carla could not restrict herself to three regular meals without feeling deprived.

As a child, Carla had been abused. She "waited" to get through childhood, promising herself she could have and do whatever she wanted. As an adult, she refused to constrain her food choices and hated being told what to do. (She had a little five-year-old inside, who was stomping her feet and refusing to compromise.)

Even though I've been waiting my whole life to get through childhood, so I can have whatever I want and do whatever I want...

Even though I HATE being told what to do...no diet is going to tell me what to do...

Even though I don't like to wait...I want to have it right away...and I'm afraid it won't be enough...

Even though I refuse to be "without," even though it's costing me...

Reminder Phrases:

I don't like to wait.

I have to have it right now.

I might not get through the day.

It won't be enough.

I refuse to be without.

I WILL have what I want.

No one is going to tell me what to do.

You can't make me.

At this point, Carla began to describe her childhood abuse, in which she endured numerous instances of being hit herself and also witnessing her brother being hit by her father. Like many trauma victims, Carla would dissociate during the abuse. "I could disconnect my head off my shoulders," she recalled. "I could leave my body and be really still."

Carla knew that "being really still" was the key to her survival. As much as the abuse hurt, struggling or running would have made it worse. Carla's survival mode was to imagine that all of her weight was going down into her feet. Being "weighted down" would keep her from running and minimize the abuse. She even imagined herself wearing leaded boots that would anchor her.

Carla also believed that if she kept a layer of padding (extra weight) on her body, the abuse would be less painful. If the padding wasn't there, she would have no protection. As an adult, she still thought that the "padding" kept her safe. It didn't feel safe to lose weight.

Carla was incredibly relieved to make these connections. After addressing several of the specific abuse events from her childhood, her binge eating is greatly decreased, and she can now eat three healthy meals per day without feeling rebellious.

I have worked with Carla for 12 sessions. She was astounded by her progress using EFT compared to traditional therapy. Her question to me at the end of this session was, "How can I have accomplished more in 12 EFT sessions than I have spending thousands of dollars and hundreds of hours in traditional therapy?" That's EFT!

❋ ❋ ❋

While this next article by Dr. Solomon has a binge-eating focus, its concepts can be used for many kinds of success blocks. As she explains, "Since our work together, Johnna has gone from binge eating several times per month to zero binge eating for the past two months. Success! No reverting back to old patterns. This process, of course, can be repeated for other avenues of success."

Treating Self-sabotage Eliminates Binge Eating
by Dr. Carol Solomon

My client, Johnna, was incredibly capable, but she found herself continuously sabotaging her success. She would get close to her goal, whether it was weight loss or creative endeavors, and suddenly revert back to old behavior.

This was particularly obvious with her binge eating problem. Several times per month she would go "over the edge" and eat everything in sight. She made several attempts to overcome this problem but, alas, she reverted back every time.

It was as though a wet blanket was thrown on her drive toward her goal. Her inner critic would then show up, and she would have self-talk such as, "Who do you think you are?" Johnna did not believe that she was allowed to be successful in anything, binge-eating control included.

Johnna recognized her pattern of self-sabotage. There seemed to be some fear of success, but she couldn't identify the source of the problem. Keeping in mind her lack of success with binge eating, we started with some general EFT statements:

Even though success does not feel safe, I deeply and completely accept myself.

Even though success does not feel good, I deeply love and accept myself anyway.

Even though success feels threatening, I choose to love and accept myself completely.

Then we used some general Reminder Phrases to tap around the body:

Success doesn't feel safe.

Success doesn't feel good.

Success is threatening.

Part of me doesn't want to succeed.

Who do you think you are?

I'm not allowed to have it.

Part of me doesn't want to change.

It just doesn't feel right.

At this point, Johnna remembered that whenever she was successful, her parents would no longer help her. When she learned how to bake cookies, for example, her mother was happy and relieved. She would withdraw her support and turn that responsibility over to Johnna. It made Johnna feel alone, lonely, and overwhelmed, since she was saddled with more and more adult responsibilities.

She was always expected to handle these responsibilities. It was what her parents valued in her. But for Johnna, success meant losing contact with her parents, feeling alone and unsupported.

It was such a well-entrenched, unconscious pattern that as an adult, Johnna became anxious whenever she neared success. If she lost weight, she was afraid there wouldn't be any support and that others would expect more of her.

She routinely sabotaged her success in order to feel less anxious. Yet, she felt frustrated knowing that she was repeating the same vicious cycle over and over again. It was only during EFT sessions that these patterns became clear.

Once the patterns were clear, we identified some events from her past that were clearly causing these blocks to her success. Using more EFT, we resolved the emotional aspects of those events and Johnna soon started to feel the freedom.

Since our work together, Johnna has gone from binge eating several times per month to zero binge eating for the past two months. Success! No reverting back to old patterns. This process, of course, can be repeated for other avenues of success.

❉ ❉ ❉

Once again, Dr. Solomon shows us how effective EFT can be with overeating once you find the core issues.

Is It Safe to Drop Those Pounds?
by Dr. Carol Solomon

Sue was a binge eater who seemed to sabotage herself at every turn. She tried everything and lost weight many times, only to gain it back and more. She described her eating as being "like a runaway train." She ate to relieve stress. She ate to celebrate. She ate for every emotion she ever felt. And she felt like a failure.

Sue's mother always struggled with her weight and died of lung cancer at an early age. Right before she was diagnosed, she lost 20 pounds and looked great. She stopped dieting, but continued to lose weight. Sue recalled that her mother remarked, "Gee, I stopped dieting and I'm still losing weight." But the weight loss happened because she had cancer. She died soon afterwards.

Food was comforting, but Sue wanted to feel more in control, to stop bingeing, and to use food for nutrition, not as a drug. She lived alone and felt scared at night. She was afraid of dying, of going to sleep and not waking up. Every day, she ate sensibly. Every night, she blew it. She found herself circling the pizza place, telling herself, "You're tired, you deserve it, you can start tomorrow." She was medicating herself to get to sleep.

Every time Sue started to lose weight, she got scared. She felt vulnerable. *It just didn't feel safe.* Food gave her that false sense of comfort because food and comfort were linked in her mind. Her grandmother fed her to comfort her. Her mother died when she lost weight. Part of her was afraid to lose weight, even though consciously, she desired it.

Strong associations can impact our behavior. In Sue's mind, food was associated with comfort and safety. Weight loss was associated with fear, loss and death. She was afraid that if she lost weight, something terrible would happen. Losing weight wasn't safe.

Binge eating is a coping behavior—a reaction to life's problems. It's easy to feel consumed by your emotions. Binge eaters often get into circular patterns of not sleeping well, overworking and feeling tired, and then being more vulnerable to bingeing.

Fears tend to surface at night, so Sue tapped at night whenever she felt afraid and/or felt the urge to binge. She tapped on her feelings about losing her mom, her fears of losing her co-workers, her fear of not waking up. Within three nights, she was able to feel more calm and relaxed and get more sleep, thus interrupting the vicious cycle. When her fears were resolved, there was no need to soothe herself with food. Within a week, she was no longer bingeing.

It's been a few months now and Sue's last note to me simply said, "I can't remember the last time I binged, and I've managed to lose 10 pounds in the process."

✳ ✳ ✳

Brazilian therapist Sonia Novinsky spends her time using EFT and affirmations to go straight for the emotional causes—and in the following bulimia case there are many of them, as you will see. The result? A complete cessation of symptoms. What else would you expect when you have eradicated the cause?

You will note in Sonia's message that English is not her first language. Further, she had to write in a hurried state between appointments. Nonetheless, her conviction, caring, and skill come across quite clearly. Since writing this report, she has worked with at least five other clients with compulsive eating disorders, and all were treated successfully, with no recurring symptoms. How many eating disorder specialists can say that? Hopefully, Sonia's message will find its way into eating disorder clinics around the world and initiate healing at new levels.

Don't you just love it when one voice from a far-away land can bring healing to many?

Bulimia in Brazil

by Sonia Novinsky

Shelly is my bulimic client. She is a personal trainer, 34 years old, married, with one child.

I worked with her for three months, once a week, from June to September, 1999. Then she came till January once a month, only for checking, and the symptoms didn't came back.

Symptoms started in her early twenties (she got married at 24). From menstruation phase (11 years old) till age 24, she wasn't allowed to date, go out, take a shower, or dress herself beautifully. All day in the bedroom, crying most of the time, feeling shame of being fat. Almost no memories of these years. Very severe depression after delivery of her child.

When she arrived she was taking Reductil (a weight-loss prescription drug) and two anti-depressants, Prozac and Tryptanol. When she left she was free from these drugs.

Symptoms: She ate compulsively, till no place was left in the stomach, mainly in the evening. Then she vomited or ran 10 to 30 km (6 to 19 miles) for sweating out all the calories.

Then she started eating again. Was obsessive about losing weight. Not fat at all. Three lipoaspiration surgeries in the belly and in the buttocks. In addition, compulsive shopping until bankrupt.

Using EFT and affirmations, I helped her work with the following family issues.

1. Her mother has been very sick since adolescence with a very rare kind of leprosy, no cure available. Very disagreeable spots in the skin. Shelly never felt permission to develop her own femininity. Guilty of being beautiful.

2. Grandmother living in the same house, taking care of Shelly's mother and the children. A very authoritarian person, violent, seducer and intrusive (including in sexual issues) — feelings of hate and guilt. The grandmother used to say that Shelly and her brother were responsible for the spots on their mother's body. Shelly yelled, "You

are not my mother!" She felt guilty all the time and wore only male clothes.

3. Her father (a compulsive eater, maybe bulimic also, she thinks) felt in a trap, He didn't know the mother had this terrible leprosy before marriage. Violent conflicts at home all the time. She feels her father at the same time looks at her in a sensual way, and with contempt. Once she put her hand on his shoulder and he screamed, "I am not your boyfriend!" Very ambivalent situation. Feelings: Shame, guilt, and a lot of passion and rage.

   Whenever she felt better, thinner, or beautiful, and her father said a compliment, like, "You look beautiful today," this immediately triggered a deep tension and the compulsion to eat and throw up the food. And she start gaining weight again while feeling that food is in a bad place in the body and has to be thrown away in some way (through vomiting or aerobic activity). Feelings: Fear of being beautiful, fear of not being able to set limits, fear of becoming a whore.

4. Marriage issues: Limits issues with her husband and his family.

Results:

1. She is more comfortable when visiting her mother and father. No tension felt anymore.

2. No compulsion at all (zero on the 0-to-10 scale) for buying and eating food. No need to eliminate

food from the body or to fast (she used before to fast some days to eliminate food).

3. She started wearing more feminine clothes. Shame and guilt = zero

4. She now can look in the mirror and love herself. Rage = zero

5. She is now setting limits and protecting herself from her husband's intrusive family. Being able to say, "I don't want you here today," for example.

6. More healthy relationship with job and career, attracting more stable clients.

[*My comment:* Six months later, Sonia sent the following update. While Shelly still had no trace of her bulimic reaction, she developed other eating/weight responses to recent events in her life. This should come as no surprise, especially given Shelly's difficult childhood. While Shelly has freedom on some things, there are now new issues that are begging for attention. Here is Sonia's message. Her English, while not perfect, carries within it abundant evidence of her skill and caring.]

Shelly came today. Very interesting.

Shopping compulsion: Never more.

Bulimic reactions: Never more.

Job as personal trainer: Seven clients per day (earning money).

But something happened with her eating compulsion.

After our last session, I called asking for permission to tell her story to a magazine that invited me for an interview. She agreed immediately, but this phone call triggered a very anxious feeling: *"I can't deal with a success. I can't sustain a success, I prefer to leave forever, there is no durable success for me."*

After this she never tapped again and never called me back again. She just forgot me. It's a pattern. Whenever she has a success with someone or receives some public recognition, and she gave several examples, she leaves immediately and cuts the person off.

Then she was involved in a big stress in February because her husband went bankrupt, and she had some serious dental work. When this occurred, she gained 3 kilograms, or 7 pounds. She had been a constant 62 kilograms or 136 pounds since our treatment. Now she felt some compulsion but not a bulimic reaction. She is working very hard and has no time to indulge in a big compulsion!

I notice now a dissociation: A part of her wants to be 58–60 kilograms (127–132 pounds). Another part still can't sustain victory or success.

We will start another piece of treatment. She will pay me only if she maintains 58 kilograms (127 pounds) for a while.

Although some core issues remained untreated, including a critical one that allowed her to sabotage our connection and EFT, the bulk of our previous work is fine. She never threw up food anymore, never went to a mall to buy things on impulse, and she is very responsible in money issues, earning and sustaining her house practically alone now.

[*My comment:* In this second follow-up, Sonia completes her report.]

I think my work with Shelly just finished today. She is feeling great. I will see her next week for the last time. Today she told me some important feelings she had last week that give evidence she is OK:

1. She is dressing herself in a feminine way almost everyday. Previously she wore men's clothes because of her shame.

2. Someone said, *"How thin you are!"* And she liked this and did not feel the urge to eat compulsively after that.

3. Her mother said, *"The way you are using your hair is like whores use it!"* And she smiled and translated for herself, *"I am beautiful, my hair is beautiful, and I don't feel ashamed or guilty."*

4. She is in a wonderful moment with her husband. And when they were having sex and he passed his hands over her body, she felt appreciation for her weight, which is something really new for her.

5. Just before menstruation, when she normally succumbed to cravings, she realized she could eat a piece of chocolate and then stop immediately.

6. During the weekend (when she used to eat a lot), she now talks to herself as follows, *"I want to have the pleasure of being skinny, so I will not have the*

pleasure of eating a lot now. I can postpone my pleasure." And she is playing with this new possibility in her life, to postpone pleasure sometimes. For example, she postponed the pleasure of reading a magazine she wanted to read as soon as she bought it, choosing instead to read it later while alone and in a peaceful moment, and so on.

7. She was alone Saturday night (a good moment for the compulsion) and she didn't feel any emptiness inside. She called some friends, drank a juice, watched a soap opera, and fell asleep. EFT has completely changed her life.

❀ ❀ ❀

Eating disorders such as bulimia are often complex and may take many sessions to resolve. Once in a while, however, we get a "one-session wonder" and major progress occurs within one hour. Such is the case in this report by Therese Baumgart. Note how Therese gets to the emotional drivers behind the disorder.

Two-Year Bulimia Problem
Improves in One Hour

by Therese Baumgart

Linda is a vibrant, athletic career woman and mother. Prior to her first appointment she told me on the phone that she had a food issue, but she was not specific. When she arrived in my office she said she had never told anybody before, but she had been bingeing and purging for two years. What began as a twice-a-month event had now increased to twice a week. As she related this problem, and through most of our session, Linda was very emotional. I used her information and often her exact wording to construct her EFT Setups and Reminder Phrases. Linda mirrored my tapping on herself as we worked together while saying:

Even though I feel ashamed and disgusted with myself, I deeply and completely accept myself.

This is a secret I never told anyone…

I'm so humiliated and embarrassed…

Bingeing and purging is my secret, and I'm so ashamed…

If they found out, they would say it's so disgusting…

They would say, Linda, how could you do that?

The worst thing in the world is for them to find out…

They would criticize, reject, and judge me harshly…

As Linda was getting ready to leave, she mentioned that she was most tempted to binge and purge in the afternoons. So for additional support during the two weeks between our first and second sessions, I recommended that every morning before starting her daily activities, Linda "set up the day" with EFT.

I also told Linda to follow her own thoughts and use them for her EFT Setups and statements.

I believe that part of Linda's rapid progress is due to her high motivation to help herself and her complete acceptance and enthusiasm for EFT. She started our first session extremely distressed and crying and ended the session with a huge confident smile, saying that she felt "wonderful."

Two weeks later, Linda reported that she had not had any bulimia episodes and had been faithful in doing her set-up-the-day phrases as well as tapping daily on whatever issues came up. She had even attended her family's Thanksgiving dinner and felt a little too full but had used EFT to handle the situation successfully.

During her second appointment we identified a core-issue incident from her childhood involving her mother, which echoed some of the emotions and thoughts around her bulimia. We used EFT to release these related core issues from 10 down to 0. Linda is now optimistic and confident about her continued success, and so am I.

After her first session, Linda wrote, "As I reflect on the last one and a half weeks since we met, the overall sense I have is that the torment is gone from my relationship with food. Before I came to see you and had my first EFT session, I had definite feelings of inadequacy, hopelessness, and helplessness about bingeing and my weight. I did not realize the amount of shame I felt about my actions in the area of bingeing.

"I have to say for the first time," she concluded, "that I feel like I have a healthy home inside myself, a place I can go, through tapping, that soothes, comforts, and cares for me and my feelings. I hear the torment and I 'go home' to the comfort and compassion of the tapping session. It is truly a relief and grace for me. I look forward to our next session."

❀ ❀ ❀

In this next report from Aileen Nobles, one professionally applied session brought relief to a client who went from bingeing and purging twice a day to zero occurrences in the following six weeks.

A Bulimia "One-Session Wonder"

by Aileen Nobles

About a month ago a client came to me with major anxiety issues. She had reverted back to a bulimic pattern that she has had on and off since she was a teen. She's in her late thirties now. She fully understood the dangers of this behavior but had been eating and purging twice a day for the last four months.

She was very clear as to when it first started. Her mother had been at a birthday party with her and she had eaten too much cake and didn't feel so well. Her mother told her that if she could make herself throw up she would feel better. She did…and, indeed, she felt better!

She also said that she was teased at school about her body, yet if she looked at a photo of herself at school, she saw that she wasn't fat.

We did a basic round on:

Even though my mother suggested I throw up if I've eaten too much, I can still completely accept myself.

Even though I'm trying to throw up all of my anxiety, fear, and ugly feelings about myself, It's OK. I can still completely accept myself.

My mother didn't always suggest the best things for me, and throwing up after eating is one of them.

I chose to use "is" instead of "was" to bring these events into present time. We did another round on:

My mother drank too much and didn't feel good about herself so she put a lot of pressure on me to look and perform a certain way.

The client had been a child actor.

I then suggested that she relax and imagine all of the negative images that came from her mother and the children at school. We started tapping on her issues of anxiety and fear and brought those levels way down.

We went back to:

Even though I can't get rid of my fear and anxiety by throwing it up, I deeply and completely accept myself.

Even though it would be much better if I don't overeat in the first place...

We went on to issues of not liking the way she looks. I asked her to tell me what she disliked and liked about her appearance. She focused on disliking her legs, thighs, and behind. She suddenly remembered very vividly being called "fat ass" in school. It still triggered a strong reaction as she thought about it. We tapped on:

Even though I have a fat ass, I don't need to throw up.

I threw in a reframe about the size of Serena Williams' rear end and how it was revered by thousands. (My client actually has a nice fairly small curved rear end.)

It's been six weeks now and, so far, she has had no desire to binge. Please recall that, before EFT, she was bingeing and purging twice a day. She taps on herself for the anxiety and fear. I just love it when EFT works this well.

❊ ❊ ❊

EFT Glossary

The following terms have specific meanings in EFT. They are referred to in some of the reports included here and are often mentioned in EFT reports.

Acupoints. Acupuncture points that are sensitive points along the body's meridians. Acupoints can be stimulated by acupuncture needles or, in acupressure, by massage or tapping. EFT is an acupressure tapping technique.

Art of Delivery. The sophisticated presentation of EFT that uses imagination, intuition, and humor to quickly discover and treat the underlying causes of pain and other problems. The art of delivery goes far beyond basic EFT.

Aspects. "Issues within issues," or different facets or pieces of a problem that are related but separate. When new aspects appear, EFT can seem to stop working. In truth, the original EFT treatment continues to work while the new aspect triggers a new set of symptoms. In some cases, many aspects of a situation or problem each require their own EFT treatment. In others, only a few do.

Basic Recipe (also known as Mechanical EFT). EFT's basic protocol, which consists of tapping on the Karate Chop point or Sore Spot while saying three times, "Even though I have this ___[problem]___ , I fully and complete accept myself" (Setup Phrase), followed by three rounds of tapping the Sequence of EFT acupoints in order, with an appropriate Reminder Phrase. See also Full Basic Recipe.

Borrowing Benefits. When you tap with or on behalf of another person, your own situation improves, even though you aren't tapping for your own situation. This happens in one-on-one sessions, in groups, and when you perform surrogate or proxy tapping. The more you tap for others, the more your own life improves.

Chasing the Pain. After applying EFT, physical discomforts can move to other locations and/or change in intensity or quality. A headache described as a sharp pain behind the eyes at an intensity of 8 might shift to a dull throb at the back of the head at an intensity of 7 (or 9, or 3, or any other intensity level). Moving pain is an indication that EFT is working. Keep "chasing the pain" with EFT and it will usually go to 0 or some low number. In the process, emotional issues behind the discomforts are often successfully treated.

Chi. Vital energy that flows through and around every living being. Chi is said to regulate spiritual, emotional, mental, and physical balance and to be influenced by *yin* (the receptive, feminine force) and *yang* (the active masculine force). These forces, which are complementary opposites, are in constant motion. When yin and yang are balanced, they work together with the natural flow of chi to help the body achieve and maintain health. Chi moves through the body along invisible pathways, or channels, called meridians. Traditional Chinese medicine identifies twenty meridians through which chi flows or circulates to all parts of the body. Acupoints along the meridians can be stimulated to improve the flow of chi and, in EFT, to resolve emotional issues.

Choices Method. Dr. Patricia Carrington's method for inserting positive statements and solutions into Setup and Reminder Phrases.

Core Issues. Deep, important underlying emotional imbalances, usually created in response to traumatic events. A core issue is truly the crux of the problem, its root or heart. Core issues are not always obvious but careful detective work can often uncover them and, once discovered, they can be broken down into specific events and handled routinely with EFT.

Full Basic Recipe. A four-step treatment consisting of Setup phrase, Sequence (tapping on acupoints in order), 9-Gamut Procedure, and Sequence. This was the original EFT protocol.

Generalization Effect. When related issues are neutralized with EFT, they often take with them issues that are related in the person's mind. In this way, several issues can be resolved even though only one is directly treated.

Global. Though the term "global" usually refers to something universal or experienced worldwide, in EFT it refers to problems stated in vague and nonspecific terms, especially in Setup Phrases.

Intensity Meter. The 0-to-10 scale that measures pain, discomfort, anger, frustration, and every other physical or emotional symptom. Intensity can also be indicated with gestures, such as hands held close together (small discomfort) or wide apart (large discomfort).

Mechanical EFT. See Basic Recipe.

Meridians. Invisible channels or pathways through which energy *(chi)* flows in the body. The eight primary meridians pass through five pairs of vital organs, and twelve secondary meridians network to the extremities. The basic premise of EFT is that the cause of every negative emotion and most physical symptoms is a block or disruption in the flow of chi along one or more of the meridians.

Movie Technique, or Watch the Movie Technique. In this process, you review in your mind, as though it were a movie, a bothersome specific event. When intensity comes up, stop and tap on that intensity. When the intensity subsides, continue in your mind with the story. This method has been a mainstay in the toolbox of many EFT practitioners. It may be the most-used EFT technique. For a full description, see www. EFTUniverse.com/tutorial/tutorcthree.htm

Personal Peace Procedure. An exercise in which you clear problems and release core issues by writing down, as quickly as possible, as many bothersome events from your life that you can remember. Try for at least fifty, or a hundred. Give each event a title, as though it is a book or movie. When the list is complete, begin tapping on the largest issues. Eliminating at least one uncomfortable memory per day (a very conservative schedule) removes at least ninety unhappy events in three months. If you work through two or three per day, it's 180 or 270. For details, see www. EFTUniverse.com/tutorial/tutormthirteen.htm.

Reminder Phrase. A word, phrase, or sentence that helps the mind focus on the problem being treated. It is used in combination with acupoint tapping.

Setup Phrase, or Setup. An opening statement said at the beginning of each EFT treatment that defines and helps neutralize the problem. In EFT, the standard Setup Phrase is "Even though I have this _____, I fully and completely accept myself."

Story Technique, or Tell the Story Technique. Narrate or tell out loud the story of a specific event dealing with trauma, grief, anger, and so on, and stop to tap whenever the story becomes emotionally intense. Each of the stopping points represents another aspect of the issue that, on occasion, will take you to even deeper issues. This technique is similar to the Movie Technique, except that in the Movie Technique, you simply watch past events unfold in your mind. In the Story Technique, you describe them out loud.

Surrogate or Proxy Tapping. Tapping on yourself on behalf of another person. The person can be present or not. Another way to perform surrogate or proxy tapping is to substitute a photograph, picture, or line drawing for the person and tap on that.

Tail-Enders. The "yes, but" statements that create negative self-talk. When you state a goal or affirmation, tail-enders point the way to core issues.

Tearless Trauma Technique. This is another way of approaching an emotional problem in a gentle way. It involves having the client guess as to the emotional intensity of a past event rather than painfully relive it mentally.

Writings on Your Walls. Limiting beliefs and attitudes that result from cultural conditioning or family attitudes, these are often illogical and harmful yet very strong subconscious influences.

Yin and Yang. See Chi.

Appendix A:
The Full Basic Recipe

Although the shortcut version of EFT that's described throughout this book works well almost all of the time, the original version of EFT, which is described in *The EFT Manual*, contains additional features that are sometimes necessary. I recommend that everyone who's learning EFT become familiar with the full Basic Recipe, which includes tapping points on the fingers as well as the 9 Gamut Procedure. After you master the full Basic Recipe, feel free to put the finger points and the 9 Gamut Procedure on the shelf. As long as you obtain good results from the shortcut version, save time by using it—but if you feel stuck, try a few rounds of the original process.

Ingredient #1: The Setup

The full Basic Recipe begins with the Setup Phrase:

Even though I have this _____, I deeply and completely accept myself.

While reciting the Setup Phrase, either tap on the Karate Chop point or massage your Sore Spot.

The Sore Spot (described below) is not part of the shortcut EFT method described in this book, but it can be substituted for the Karate Chop point at the beginning of any EFT session. Here's how to find it.

The Sore Spot

There are two Sore Spots and it doesn't matter which one you use. They are located in the upper left and right portions of the chest.

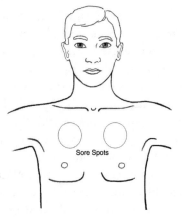

The Sore Spot.

Go to the base of the throat about where a man would knot his tie. Poke around in this area and you will find a U shaped notch at the top of your sternum (breastbone). From the top of that notch go down 2 or 3 inches toward your navel and sideways 2 or 3 inches to your left (or right). You should now be in the upper left (or right) portion of your chest. If you press vigorously in that area (within a 2-inch radius) you will find a spot that feels sore or tender. This happens because lymphatic congestion occurs there. When you rub it, you disperse that congestion. Fortunately, after a few episodes the congestion is all dispersed and the soreness goes away. Then you can rub it with no discomfort whatsoever.

I don't mean to overplay the soreness you may feel. You won't feel massive, intense pain by rubbing this Sore Spot. It is certainly bearable and should cause no undue discomfort. If it does, then lighten up your pressure a little.

Also, if you've had some kind of operation in that area of the chest or if there's any medical reason whatsoever why you shouldn't be probing around in that specific area then *switch to the other side.* Both sides are equally effective. In any case, if there is any doubt, consult your health practitioner before proceeding or simply tap the Karate Chop point instead.

Ingredient #2: The Sequence

The Sequence involves tapping on the Eyebrow, Side of Eye, Under Eye, Under Nose, Chin, Collarbone, Under Arm, and Below Nipple points.

The **Below Nipple** point is a newer addition to the full sequence. It was originally left out because it's in an awkward position for ladies while in social situations (restaurants, etc.) as well as in workshops. Even though the EFT results have been superb without it, I include it now for completeness. For men, it is one inch below the nipple. For ladies, it's where the under-skin of the breast meets the chest wall. Some call it the "underwire" point on an underwire bra. This point is abbreviated **BN** for **B**elow Nipple.

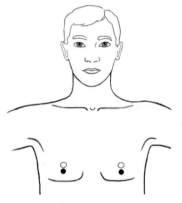

Below the Nipple (**BN**).

In addition, the Sequence in the full Basic Recipe includes the following finger points:

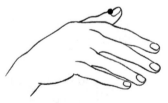

Thumb (**Th**) Point.

Thumb: On the outside edge of your thumb at a point even with the base of the thumbnail. This point is abbreviated **Th** for **Thumb**.

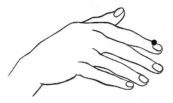

The Index Finger (**IF**) Point.

Index Finger: On the side of your index finger (the side facing your thumb) at a point even with the base of the fingernail. This point is abbreviated **IF** for Index Finger.

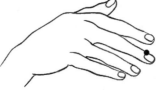

The Middle Finger (**MF**) Point.

Middle Finger: On the side of your middle finger (the side closest to your thumb) at a point even with the base of the fingernail. This point is abbreviated **MF** for Middle Finger.

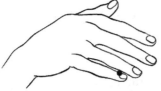

The Baby Finger (**BF**) Point.

Baby Finger: On the inside of your baby finger (the side closest to your thumb) at a point even with the base of the fingernail. This point is abbreviated **BF** for **B**aby **F**inger.

You may have noticed that the Sequence does not include the Ring Finger. However, some include it for convenience, and this does not interfere with EFT's effectiveness.

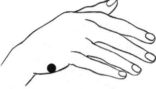

The Karate Chop (**KC**) Point.

Karate Chop: The last point is the Karate Chop point, which can also be used at the beginning of the Setup.

Thus, the complete Sequence consists of the following EFT points, which are tapped while one repeats a reminder phrase that describes the problem, such as "This headache" or "This fear of heights."

EB = Beginning of the **E**ye**B**row

SE = **S**ide of the **E**ye

UE = **U**nder the **E**ye

UN = **U**nder the **N**ose

Ch = **Ch**in

CB = Beginning of the **C**ollar**B**one

UA = **U**nder the **A**rm

BN = **B**elow the **N**ipple

Th = **Th**umb

IF = **I**ndex **F**inger

MF = **M**iddle **F**inger

BF = **B**aby **F**inger

KC = **K**arate **C**hop

Ingredient #3: The 9 Gamut Procedure

The 9 Gamut Procedure is perhaps the most bizarre looking process within EFT. Its purpose is to fine-tune" the brain, which it does so via some eye movements, humming, and counting. Through connecting nerves, certain parts of the brain are stimulated when the eyes are moved. Likewise, the right side of the brain (the creative side) is engaged when you hum a song and the left side (the digital side) is engaged when you count.

The 9 Gamut Procedure is a 10-second process in which nine "brain stimulating" actions are performed while one continuously taps on one of the body's energy points—the Gamut point. It has been found, after years of experience, that this routine can add efficiency to EFT and hasten your progress towards emotional freedom, especially when *sandwiched* between two trips through the Sequence.

One way to help memorize the Basic Recipe is to look at it as though it is a ham sandwich. The Setup is the preparation for the ham sandwich and the sandwich itself consists of two slices of bread (The Sequence) with the ham, or middle portion, as the 9 Gamut Procedure.

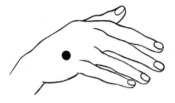

The Gamut Point.

To do the 9 Gamut Procedure, you must first locate the Gamut point. It is on the back of either hand and is 1/2 inch behind the midpoint between the knuckles at the base of the ring finger and the little finger.

If you draw an imaginary line between the knuckles at the base of the ring finger and little finger and consider that line to be the base of an equilateral triangle whose other sides converge to a point (apex) in the direction of the wrist, then the Gamut point would be located at the apex of the triangle. With the index finger of your tapping hand, feel for a small indentation on the back of your tapped hand near the base of the little finger and ring finger. There is just enough room there to tap with the tips of your index and middle fingers.

Next, you must perform nine different steps while tapping the Gamut point continuously. These 9 Gamut steps are:

1. Eyes closed.

2. Eyes open.

3. Eyes down hard right while holding the head steady.

4. Eyes down hard left while holding the head steady.

5. Roll the eyes in a circle as though your nose is at the center of a clock and you are trying to see all the numbers in order.

6. Roll the eyes in a circle in the reverse direction.

7. Hum two seconds of a song (I usually suggest "Happy Birthday").

8. Count rapidly from 1 to 5.

9. Hum two seconds of a song again.

Note that these nine actions are presented in a certain order and I suggest that you memorize them in the order given. However, you can mix the order up if you wish so long as you do all nine of them *and* you perform the last three together as a unit. That is, you hum for two seconds, then count, then hum the song again, in that order. Years of experience have proven this to be important.

Also, note that for some people humming "Happy Birthday" causes resistance because it brings up memories of unhappy birthdays. In this case, you can either use EFT on those unhappy memories and resolve them or you can side-step this issue for now by substituting some other song.

Ingredient #4: The Sequence (again)

The fourth and last ingredient in the Basic Recipe is another trip through The Sequence, including the finger points.

As in the shortcut Basic Recipe, check for any remaining discomfort, in which case you'll do another round of EFT tapping using a modified Setup Phrase:

> *Even though I still have some of this* _____*, I deeply and completely accept myself.*

You will add "remaining" to the Reminder Phrases as you tap through the complete Sequence.

For perspective, I conducted this process one afternoon in Chicago for an audience of 500 people and 499 reported impressive results. However, this does not represent a guarantee. Your results may vary from this and there's a small possibility that you may not experience any benefits at all.

Q: Are there any cautions regarding this process?

A: While Easy EFT is relatively gentle and most people fly right through it with ease, it is possible that you may open up some stressful issues. Further, about 3 or 4 percent of the population (my estimate) have such frail emotional or physical issues that they should not attempt any healing aid on their own. Such attempts could lead to stress and unwanted results. Accordingly, you are advised to consult a qualified health professional before proceeding with this method.

Helpful Tips for Getting the Most Out of Easy EFT

Watch the EFT sessions on the web. This will acquaint you with the basic tapping points and make it easier for you to tap along.

- You do not have to read *The EFT Manual* to benefit from Easy EFT.

- You may find that the EFT sessions vary the method a bit and add new tapping points from time to time. These variations represent sophistications within EFT that are not necessary for you to understand for now. Any benefits they may provide will be automatically integrated within your Easy EFT results. Just tap along.

- **At first, you may find the tapping pace in the sessions to be too fast for you to follow along.** That's OK, just do your best. The process can still help you even if you miss a tapping point here or there. Eventually, you will get used to the process and the pace will be easy to follow.

Spend quality time with your list of issues and their 0-to-10 intensities because they are the foundation of this process. Don't just throw down two or three issues and guess at their 0-to-10 ratings.

- For your list, go back to childhood and pick up every anger, guilt, fear, etc. issue you can recall. Run through them mentally to see what **current** 0-to-10 intensities they bring up, not the way you felt when it happened. Then take an inventory of your body and list every pain or other physical symptom or disease you can find. List everything and don't skip something just because you think it is too big or "impossible."

- If you can't find a 0-to-10 intensity, that's OK. Just estimate what the number should be. It's amazing how accurate such estimates tend to be. The mere fact that you remembered an issue means you have some sort of charge on it, albeit possibly repressed. These can be helped by Easy EFT.

- List as many issues as you want. The more, the merrier. Fifty is better than ten because this gives Easy

Appendix B:
Easy EFT

Now I would like to introduce you to a fast, effective, and effortless way to learn EFT. It's literally as easy as watching a video and tapping along with it. You can use one of the many EFT videos at www.EFTUniverse.com for this purpose.

The Easy EFT technique may be the most important advancement in the healing field since EFT was first introduced. It puts the essence of this powerful process within easy reach of everyone.

Here are its three simple steps.

1. Identify the issues.

Write down a list of your issues, or the things you would like to improve, and rank their current intensities on a scale of 0-to-10. For example:

Neck pain: 7   Anxiety: 5   Emotional Overeating: 9

You can also tap for specific things that bother you, such as:

Angry at the clerk who was rude to me yesterday: 8

Upset about my son's accident last week: 7

Disappointed with myself for gaining five pounds this month: 9

Really hurt by my friend's criticism: 10

2. Tap along.

Fast-forward the video until you come to a tapping session. Then simply tap along as though you were the client on the screen. It doesn't matter which sessions you choose or whether they address your issues directly. Your system will empathize with the story and automatically target your issues behind the scenes.

3. Check your results.

Revisit your list of issues and write down their new 0-to-10 intensities. You should notice some improvement each time. The more sessions you tap along with, the better your results.

That's it!

But for best results, review the *Questions and Answers* and *Helpful Tips* below.

Questions and Answers about Easy EFT

Q: How was Easy EFT discovered?

A: I first discovered this process after EFT practitioners repeatedly told me that their personal issues improved as a result of tapping along with their clients. The first example occurred when I learned that someone's thyroid function improved. Next I learned that a fear of driving over bridges vanished. And then I got a barrage of reports regarding major improvements in fears, anxieties, anger, and trauma as well as a long list of physical symptoms.

But what's astonishing about this is that the EFT practitioners weren't tapping for their own issues—they were tapping along with their clients for seemingly different issues. This is a stunning discovery and means that our systems have the intelligence to "borrow benefits" and draw parallels from someone else's session. I find this happens with great regularity and, with Easy EFT, the same thing can happen for you.

Q: Why does Easy EFT work so well?

A: As you tap along with the authentic people featured on our videos, your system finds similarities between your issues and the ones being addressed on stage, *and you don't even have to know what they are!* This often happens in the background and allows the impressive meridian-balancing feature of EFT to go to work. It's a delight to use because it automatically injects the principles of EFT into something everyone enjoys doing …watching television.

Q: Can I really benefit from a session that deals with someone else's issue?

A: Yes! It's done all the time. If a housewife, for example, taps along with a session involving a war veteran's grief, fear, guilt, anger, and trauma, her system will bring up *her own* experiences of the same emotions. Tuning into someone else's issues this way is a natural thing to do and is commonly known as empathy. Easy EFT can then address these emotions and whatever physical symptoms might be associated with them.

Sometimes you might be aware that these issues are surfacing and you may feel some discomfort. Other times, things are being addressed in the background, outside of your awareness. How will you know if you are making progress? By assessing the 0-to-10 intensities as you persistently use Easy EFT.

Q: What should I expect?

A: Properly done, many of your results should range from "clearly improved" to "completely resolved." I cannot tell you in advance which of your issues will show the most improvement, but I can say that the more sessions you tap along with, the better your results can be over time.

Many people report much less emotional baggage and the reduction (or elimination) of severe physical symptoms, such as pain, allergies, addictive cravings, and so on. While I would expect that consistency will bring you great rewards, this does not mean that every issue will be resolved or improved.

Obviously, you cannot expect Easy EFT to be as thorough as OFFICIAL EFT. Some results may come right away, while others may take a while. Accordingly, anytime you want faster results, you can visit our website for a Certified EFT Practitioner, or learn OFFICIAL EFT yourself. Otherwise, persistence and patience will often pay off in a big way.

For perspective, I conducted this process one afternoon in Chicago for an audience of 500 people and 499 reported impressive results. However, this does not represent a guarantee. Your results may vary from this and there's a small possibility that you may not experience any benefits at all.

Q: Are there any cautions regarding this process?

A: While Easy EFT is relatively gentle and most people fly right through it with ease, it is possible that you may open up some stressful issues. Further, about 3 or 4 percent of the population (my estimate) have such frail emotional or physical issues that they should not attempt any healing aid on their own. Such attempts could lead to stress and unwanted results. Accordingly, you are advised to consult a qualified health professional before proceeding with this method.

Helpful Tips for Getting the Most Out of Easy EFT

Watch the EFT sessions on the web. This will acquaint you with the basic tapping points and make it easier for you to tap along.

- You do not have to read *The EFT Manual* to benefit from Easy EFT.

- You may find that the EFT sessions vary the method a bit and add new tapping points from time to time. These variations represent sophistications within EFT that are not necessary for you to understand for now. Any benefits they may provide will be automatically integrated within your Easy EFT results. Just tap along.

- **At first, you may find the tapping pace in the sessions to be too fast for you to follow along.** That's OK, just do your best. The process can still help you even if you miss a tapping point here or there. Eventually, you will get used to the process and the pace will be easy to follow.

Spend quality time with your list of issues and their 0-to-10 intensities because they are the foundation of this process. Don't just throw down two or three issues and guess at their 0-to-10 ratings.

- For your list, go back to childhood and pick up every anger, guilt, fear, etc. issue you can recall. Run through them mentally to see what **current** 0-to-10 intensities they bring up, not the way you felt when it happened. Then take an inventory of your body and list every pain or other physical symptom or disease you can find. List everything and don't skip something just because you think it is too big or "impossible."

- If you can't find a 0-to-10 intensity, that's OK. Just estimate what the number should be. It's amazing how accurate such estimates tend to be. The mere fact that you remembered an issue means you have some sort of charge on it, albeit possibly repressed. These can be helped by Easy EFT.

- List as many issues as you want. The more, the merrier. Fifty is better than ten because this gives Easy

EFT a wider doorway through which it can provide benefits.

- Your list might look something like the chart below after a few tap-along sessions. This example is for illustration only and does not indicate what you should expect on the specific items listed. Note that some of your issues will do better than others and some may not make much progress. **You will need to look at the overall picture to properly evaluate how well Easy EFT is doing for you.**

Issue	Original 0-to-10	Session 1 0-to-10	Session 2 0-to-10	Session 3 0-to-10	Etc.
Fear of Heights	8	5	2	3	
Easily Angered	10	10	5	2	
Test Anxiety	7	7	5	7	
Knee Pain	9	2	0	0	
Digestion Problems	4	4	2	3	
Etc.					
Etc.					
Etc.					

To find the tapping sessions, browse the free videos on the www.EFTUniverse.com until you find two or more people tapping together. Then rewind back to the beginning of the session and tap along as though you were the person being helped. It doesn't matter that your issues may be different from the people on stage. You will find that their issues will bring up yours. At the core, our issues are all very similar.

Some of your results may be subtle and you may not notice them until later. Further, you may also have some pleasant "side benefits" wherein improvements occur that you weren't expecting. Here are some examples:

Uncle Joe's aggressive personality may no longer bother you.

People may say that you seem more relaxed.

Your golf game may improve.

You may sleep better.

You may enjoy your work more.

Certain memories may no longer bother you.

Physical symptoms may improve.

Read your list of issues before each tap-along session just to remind your system of what you are working on. After that, put the list aside and ignore your issues —there is no need to keep focusing on them. Leave them alone so your system can draw on its wisdom and work on your issues in the background. Just tap along and enjoy the session while Easy EFT goes to work.

Revisit your list after each tap-along session. Then go through each issue and carefully assess any changes in current intensity. Write them all down, even those that haven't changed. Then do another tap-along session and visit the list again.

Do your sessions on any schedule you like. You can do them daily, weekly, or at any time interval you choose. You can even do several per day or break them up so that you do a half session today and finish it tomorrow. It all depends on your schedule.

Get plenty of EFT sessions to work with. There are books and videos at www.EFTUniverse.com that contain one or more sessions. In combination, they offer an impressive variety of issues from which to choose, and represent a lifetime of healing possibilities for you and your family.

Take the Ideal Weight EFT support course. On www.EFTUniverse.com you'll find a web community that helps you lose weight, day by day and week by week, using a proven program that has been used by thousands of other people. You'll find more information in Appendix C.

Most Importantly...have fun with it!

EFT doesn't have to be complicated, difficult, or totally serious. You'll find plenty to laugh about in our EFT books, any EFT workshops you may attend, and your own EFT sessions at home.

For free online video demonstrations of EFT as well as a complete catalog of EFT books and DVDs, visit www.EFTUniverse.com. While there, download our free EFT starter kit, sign up for our free email newsletter, search through our newsletter archives for topics of interest to you, take a look at our online tutorials, and visit our special forums.

Appendix C: Ideal Weight EFT: The Online EFT Weight-Loss Training Program

Ideal Weight EFT is a powerful weight management system that delivers fast and measurable results. It is based on the experiences of the thousands of people who have met their weight goals with EFT. It is a proven method for resolving eating disorders such as binge eating, emotional eating, bulimia and anorexia. It has already helped thousands of people online and in person, and is supported by several scientific studies. Ideal Weight EFT supports you in defining your ideal weight, and then walks you, step by step, through a customized program designed by you and for you. It is especially effective for people who have been unsuccessful with dieting, exercise, and other methods of weight control. It takes the principles you find in the book *EFT for Weight Loss* and puts them into a practical day-by-day program.

Ideal Weight EFT is not a diet. It is a comprehensive system, based on three principles:

1. **A Simple, Natural Food Program.** The Ideal Weight EFT program helps you to use your intuition and body signals to identify and enjoy food choices that allow you to be slim—yet also to feel full, and to be alert and energetic.

2. **Emotional Self-Management.** When you are able to manage your emotions, you can more easily manage your food intake, and really enjoy the pleasures of eating. The Ideal Weigh EFT program teaches you how to use EFT in conjunction with other leading-edge techniques drawn from meditation and biofeedback, such as heart coherence and mindfulness. These techniques combine to allow you to reach your ideal weight at your own pace. The course includes subliminal audio tracks that help you to relax, to learn, and to integrate these techniques effortlessly while you sleep.

3. **Group Support.** A great strength of Ideal Weight EFT is that you're not alone. You're one of a group of like-minded people who support your goals and cheer you on. They have objectives similar to yours, and they help motivate you to stay with the program. Ideal Weight EFT has discussion groups of people who share their insights and answers with you, and help you stay on track with your chosen program. You'll make friends at Ideal Weight EFT!

Your brain is like a computer, in that you know what's in the files in your conscious mind, but you don't know what's in your subconscious. That's where the programming files are found. Subconscious urges might push you, and you translate them into the language of food: hunger and gratification. These subconsciously programmed habits then determine the quantity and type of food you consume.

This programming, however, may provide us with the wrong signals for what to eat, when to eat, and how much to eat. It may override our body's natural hunger signals, and satisfaction cues such as a feeling of fullness. Feelings such as "I am sad" or "I am angry" or "I am tired" are often misinterpreted as hunger.

For this reason, the heart of the Ideal Weight EFT program is the management of your feelings. By mastering them, you are able to hear the real messages your body is sending, and get control of the quality and quantity of what goes into your mouth.

How do you get there? You use the emotional management techniques in this course. EFT allows you to eliminate the negative thoughts and feelings that hold you back. Participants in this program discover, to their surprise, that as well as reaching their ideal weight, they often increase their confidence and self-esteem.

You can sign up for a free trial at

www.IdealWeightEFT.com

and check it out before you go any further. If you enjoy the experience, you'll enjoy becoming part of the Ideal Weight EFT community.

EFT Resources

For information about EFT, including a free downloadable Get Started package, go to www.EFTUniverse. com. On this website, you'll find thousands of case histories of people who've used EFT successfully for every conceivable problem. You'll also find practitioner listings, tutorials, books, DVDs, classes, volunteer opportunities, and other resources to allow you to get the most from EFT.

Also, see www.IdealWeightEFT.com.

Index

A world of wellness at your fingertips!

To see more books in this series of authorized EFT guides, including...

The EFT Manual
EFT for Fibromyalgia and Chronic Fatigue
EFT for the Highly Sensitive Temperament
EFT for Sports Performance
EFT for Golf
EFT for Love Relationships
EFT for Abundance
EFT for Posttraumatic Stress Syndrome
EFT for Procrastination
EFT for Back Pain

...go to www.EFTuniverse.com